Saving Babies:

The Moms2B Story

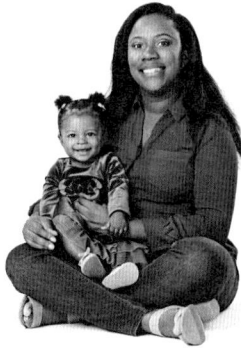

by Patricia T. Gabbe, MD, MPH
(Dr. Pat)

The Ohio State University College of Medicine
Moms2B, The Department of Obstetrics and Gynecology
395 West Twelfth Avenue, Fifth Floor
Columbus, Ohio 43210-1267

The Medical Heritage Center (MHC) is the special collections at The
Ohio State University Health Sciences Library. Proceeds from the
sale of this book support the MHC and Moms2B.

Cover, page layout and book design:
Anthony S. Baker, HSL Medical Visuals, The Ohio State University
Printing: UniPrint

Front cover: photo of Destiny Laney with her daughter Katara
taken by Bender & Bender Photography, Inc.
Back cover: Moms2B flyer, 2010

ISBN: 979-8-218-09692-2

Dedication

*I dedicate the story that follows to the families
who trusted us to teach, support and accompany them
on their journey to parenthood.*

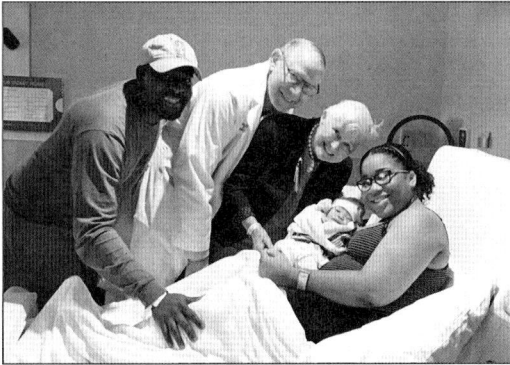

Drs. Steve and Pat Gabbe congratulate Benjamin
and Kalia Dorelien after the arrival of their son
Malachi, a Moms2B baby, in 2016.

Table of Contents

Saving Babies, Supporting Moms: The Moms2B Story

Introduction

I returned to Ohio in 2008 shocked to find persistently high rates of Black infant deaths. For every thousand Black births, fifteen infants died, more than twice the rate in white families and similar to those of white infants 40 years ago. Our Black infants died at rates seen in some of the world's poorest developing countries. I needed to understand why Ohio had such grim statistics. Even today, after more than a decade of studying Ohio's infant mortality rates and starting Moms2B, a program to alleviate the Black-white disparities, I stare in disbelief when I see Black infant death rates two to three times white infant deaths.

We have made some important strides as a state in the 14 intervening years. We have saved more babies, yet Ohio remains near the bottom of state rankings for Black infant death rates, and we still have untenable disparities, and much work to do. "We must do something," I said after spending a year on Ohio Governor Ted Strickland's infant mortality task force in 2009. Invited by Ohio's Department of Health I joined a group of 30 maternal and infant health care experts from across the state. We were charged with summarizing the causes of such high rates of infant deaths and Black-white disparities. Throughout the year we held discussion groups focused on maternal health and infant care. Our thoughtful, in-depth report listed 10 recommendations, two of which stand out: "Eliminate health disparities and promote health equity to reduce infant mortality" and "Address the effects of racism and the impact of racism on infant mortality."

Dr. Alvin Jackson, then director of the Ohio Department of Health introduced the 2009 report from the task force's work with a quote from me: *"Infant deaths are at the heart of our inadequate health care system. Why should any infant die because their mother had no health insurance before she became pregnant, had little access to treat anemia, depression, asthma, diabetes or hypertension, or to safely space her last pregnancy? Infant deaths are preventable if we realign our priorities and our financial incentives. Thank you for allowing me to be part of this process to help set Ohio on a path to better health for women and children."* [1]

Looking back, I realize that I only saw part of the picture. In the coming years, through my work with Moms2B and on related city and statewide efforts, my eyes were opened to the scope of factors that influence whether a baby will be born far too soon, or at term — whether that baby will live to see a first birthday or leave behind a grieving family, a weakened community.

Early in my long pediatric career I obtained a public health degree in administration, hoping to eventually broaden my reach from the bedside into a leadership role in medicine. In my pediatric practice I worked primarily in publicly funded clinics where I took care of Black, Hispanic and immigrant families. These parents inspired me with their love for their children and their optimism while raising children under the burden of poverty and limited resources.

Later, I worked as a medical director for academic health plans. In that role, I saw the need to prevent the emotional trauma and financial burden for families of babies born too soon, and of those who did not survive. Million-dollar premature infants with long neonatal intensive care unit stays strained our health plan budgets and strained families. We needed to help women have healthier pregnancies and fewer premature births — for their sake, for the sake of their babies and also in the interest of doing a better job from a health care business perspective.

In my days in Seattle, I had worked with Nurse Family Partnership, an evidence-based nurse home visitation program for first-time pregnant teens and women to promote healthy pregnancies and parenting. A federal Healthy Start program reached out specifically to Black families, sending social workers and community health workers into their homes. Both programs have good results and still benefit moms throughout the country, and both operate in Columbus, Ohio, where we launched Moms2B.

With that perspective in mind, one of my deepest concerns after we finished the Infant Mortality Task Force report was for the moms who already had other children and were pregnant with another. This disqualified them from Nurse Family Partnership because they serve only first-time moms. And an added obstacle for many at-risk moms and babies that was on my mind: I knew that many women and teens, for myriad reasons not always within their control, would not let visitors into their homes. And many did not have a permanent home, a challenge that the Moms2B experience later crystallized for me and for my colleagues.

I wondered, "Where do these moms turn for help? What resources do they need to prevent the delivery of a low birthweight or premature infant or a sleep-related infant death?" At the time, I was working at Nationwide Children's Hospital. The chair of my department, Dr. Mike Brady, encouraged me to identify a neighborhood where a community intervention might move the needle.

Dr. Phil Scribano, a colleague at Nationwide Children's Hospital, was a member of a faculty group studying poverty and suggested

I apply for a seed grant to investigate infant mortality in the Weinland Park area near the Ohio State campus. The faculty planned to study poverty in the neighborhood and search for solutions that could be applied broadly. We agreed that if Moms2B, the name for the concept I developed, proved beneficial and if we gained the neighborhood's trust we would stay long term, at least until we could say we eliminated the Black-white disparities in premature births and infant deaths. I knew from the start that I wanted this to be a lasting partnership between our team and the community we sought to serve — not a fleeting, unsustainable research protocol without long-term, meaningful impact.

I was excited by the confluence of their work and my passion and I delved into the epidemiology of the Weinland Park area. Using detailed birth and death records from Columbus Public Health and the state's Medicaid program, I found startling inequities. In this small area with a population of about 4,000, there were 122 births, a birth rate three times the state average. Almost 90% of the babies were born to women covered by Medicaid, indicating their incomes must be below 150% of poverty. Most concerning, 19% of the infants were born premature, at less than 37 weeks gestation, and 5% were born at less than 32 weeks, putting them at exceptionally high risk for lifelong disabilities and early death. These rates exceeded national averages at the time by two to three times. In the census tract with predominantly Black births, 22% arrived prematurely, and this was reflected in a high infant mortality rate of 16.4/1,000 live births, similar to that of developing nations with much weaker health care systems, double the U.S. average and over three times the Healthy People 2010 goal of 4.5. There were high rates of early repeat pregnancies (37%) and low rates of breastfeeding (50%). Almost all (93%) infants were born to unmarried parents many of whom didn't have a high school degree (43%).

When I told my friend and maternal-fetal medicine expert Dr. Jay Iams that I planned to start a program in Weinland Park he was concerned about high rates of violent crime in the area. He was right to worry — the neighborhood was plagued by gang activity. But, as I saw it, that and the many other obstacles to well-being in the neighborhood were exactly the reason that my work belonged there. Inevitably, in a neighborhood with so much crime, live pregnant women, new mothers and infants under tremendous stress.

From my research at Vanderbilt, I knew that stress had a significant negative impact on health and pregnancies, and likely contributed to early delivery. In Weinland Park, women were living under the stress of poverty and crime and with generational stressors dating back to slavery and carried on through structural and systemic racism.

With the decision about location made, the question that loomed for me was: "What model should we try?" I knew that nurse home visitation works for women with their first pregnancy. But for the population we wanted to reach, we needed a new model.

I believed we should base our model on reducing stress, providing healthy food and fostering early connections to the medical system. To reduce stress, should we have a "pregnancy spa" with massage, a relaxing atmosphere and healthy meals? Couple the spa with a nurse home visitor?

I knew Twinkle French Schottke, an educator and infant mental health specialist, from our participation on the board of the Council on Heathy Mothers and Babies. We became mutually disillusioned with the council's approach to focus its resources primarily on a service to schedule prenatal clinical care appointments for pregnant women with public insurance — an approach that was important but seemed to ignore the broader factors contributing to poor birth outcomes. We brainstormed what we thought might be an ideal model. Twinkle convinced me of the value of a group-based model. "If women come out of their home, meet other women, it will ease their stress, depression and anxiety," she said, already understanding the power of building a supportive community.

My seed grant application listed three aims:
- Develop and pilot a collaborative model of group prenatal care education focused on meal preparation and nutrition for low-income pregnant women in the Weinland Park neighborhood.
- Identify a trusted care coordinator for each pregnant woman during her pregnancy and this education intervention.
- Make the pilot project part of our long-term goals to implement recommendations from the Governor's Infant Mortality Task Force and improve care from preconception to pregnancy to the post-partum period to improve birth outcomes and reduce disparities in vulnerable populations.

These aims remain foundational today. But it wasn't long after the first few pregnant women walked down the stairs to the kitchen and meeting room in Grace Missionary Baptist Church in Weinland Park on Sept. 8, 2010 that we knew we had to adapt our plans. We had to respond to the lived experiences of the moms and families we hoped to serve; we knew that they would be our most valuable partners. We listened to these women's stories and shaped a model to meet their needs. And we started quickly. Within a few months, we changed from our proposed method to enroll women and teens in a national Department of Agriculture program called Expanded Food Nutrition and Education Program to a unique model that became Moms2B, a program that is now more than a decade old and continues to expand and evolve based on what we learn from the families we serve.

In the chapters that follow you will hear stories from women who were evicted while caring for newborns, who were traumatized by murders and crimes in and outside their homes. You'll hear about women who had empty refrigerators, homes without appliances and newborns in intensive care. You will hear how our moms helped each other. You will see how they began to trust us. You will hear the story of why we developed a Dads2B, and how we expanded to eight Columbus neighborhoods and beyond, to Dayton. You will see, I hope, the power of listening, of building trust and of keeping open minds and open hearts.

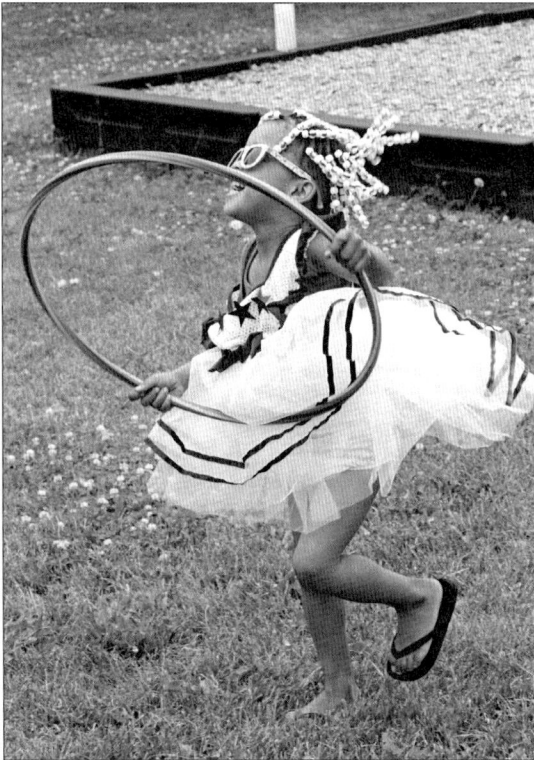

Photo: Mandy Grosko 2014

1 | Moms' Stories Take Moms2B in a New Direction

"We talk a lot about the numbers and the statistics, but this is what the real, human part looks like."

–Twinkle French Schottke, 2010, quoted in The Columbus Dispatch

On Sept. 8, 2010, we opened the front door of Grace Missionary Baptist Church in Weinland Park to welcome our first two pregnant women. We greeted them by their names, congratulated them on their pregnancies, then stepped downstairs into the church basement meeting room decorated with colorful balloons, tablecloths and streamers. It looked like a baby shower!

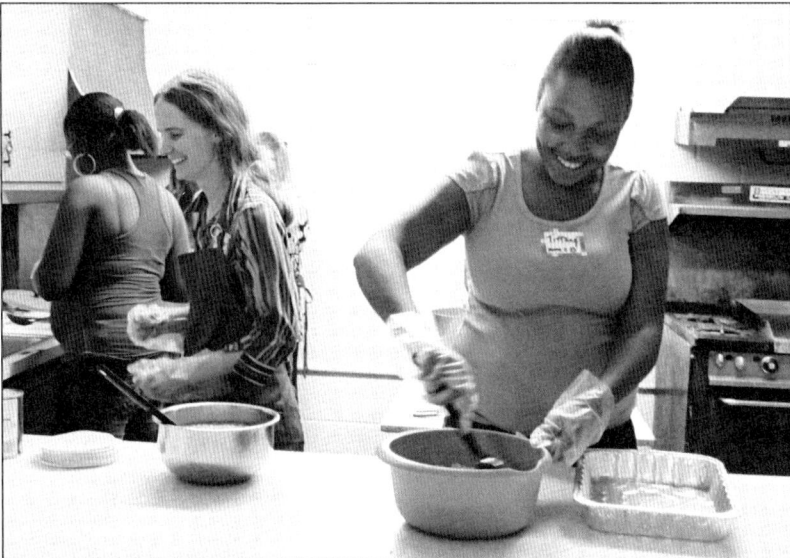

Tiffany, a Moms2B mom, helps Jen, our cooking instructor, in the kitchen at Grace Missionary Baptist Church.

Our first mom, who I will call Belinda, was scared. This was her first pregnancy and she wanted to learn more about what to expect and how to prepare for a baby. She lived in Weinland Park with her fiancé, who I will call Joseph.

On the advice of her fiancé's colleague, who knew about the upcoming launch of Moms2B, Belinda called me. I still remember that conversation. I said, "You are just in time for our new program! Come next Wednesday at 11 a.m. to Moms2B in Grace Missionary Baptist Church. You will learn about your pregnancy from nurses and doctors, and about baby care from child development experts. We will cook lunch and have fun learning together. Please come!"

I was elated and relieved. *Thank goodness, I thought, we will have at least one pregnant woman.* (For the first year I worried every week that not a single woman would come, but Twinkle French Schottke, an infant mental health specialist who co-founded Moms2B, always reassured me, saying that each two-hour session would be so engaging that moms would come and not want to leave.)

Our second mom, who I'll call Danny, had also heard about the program through a mutual colleague.

Soon after Belinda and Danny walked into our lives, we realized the program we envisioned would need to change if we hoped to address the breadth of obstacles to good health that moms in our community were facing.

In our original proposal, funded by the Ohio State Poverty Collaborative, we described a simple, structured approach to improve pregnancy outcomes. Our basic idea was sound. We would hold group prenatal education sessions focused on nutrition and the medical and psychological changes of pregnancy.

Half of our session was taught by Ohio State Extension staff following an hour-long structured cooking and nutrition curriculum developed by the U.S. Department of Agriculture for low-income pregnant women.

Other goals included encouraging breastfeeding, reducing cigarette smoking and connecting every woman to a trusted care coordinator in an existing home visiting program. After this year-long pilot with pregnant women, we expected to add preconception health education and extend Moms2B through the postpartum period, both recommendations from a recent report from the Governor's Infant Mortality Task Force.

Within a few weeks of Moms2B, Belinda shared that she and Joseph were homeless. We quickly began to learn about a complex, intertwined cluster of factors — social determinants of health, including housing, that those in health care didn't always consider, but that directly influence maternal health, birth outcomes and infant deaths.

My notes at the time tell of the cascade of events that drove this early Moms2B couple to despair.

(Belinda) is homeless. She is depressed, stressed, dressed all in black and not her usual happy, take-charge self. She and Joseph lived in a very large house in Weinland Park and their roommates helped with the electricity bills; the roommates all moved out, there was no help with the utility bills. Without electricity, heat and running water, landlords file eviction papers. They put all their belongings in storage; they are living in a motel. Joseph's father helped with the weekly $210 payment.
A few weeks before, they had put a deposit on an apartment, but there was a killing on the street and now they do not want to move there. They cannot get their deposit back.

A volunteer friend asks me if we shouldn't pitch in and give them a down payment on an apartment. We decided not at this time. During the week, Susan Colbert, from Ohio State Extension, and Twinkle try to find housing for them.

"I'm afraid the stress is bad for the baby," (Belinda) says, "and I've been smoking again." "Where is your family?" I ask her. "They are useless," she answers. She lived with a relative while her mother used drugs and her father had put a gun to her head. "I've tried to find housing but if we go to a shelter, I have to be separated from Joseph. And I don't want that."

The fastest way to find a house was through the family homeless shelter. With their connections to landlords, the shelter could house women and children within a month. However, they only accepted families. Pregnant women without children went to the general homeless shelter that had no accommodations at the time.

Fortunately, another mom in our group heard that Belinda and Joseph needed an apartment and she convinced her landlord to rent to the couple. Although Belinda and Joseph moved into a dark, cold apartment without electricity until they paid their past-due electric bill, they at least had a home.

Joyce Beatty, who was working at Ohio State at the time and later became our congresswoman, had just awarded me a $1,000 check from her charity, Fire and Focus, to help with Moms2B. We used part of it to pay the electric company to turn on the heat and lights in the couple's new apartment so their home would be ready for their baby.

Housing: an Unforeseen, Critical, Threat to Healthy Weinland Park Births

Before we submitted our detailed Moms2B proposal to Ohio State, we held extensive discussions with experts to plan the best use of our $42,800 budget. But not once had we considered or heard that women would need food and housing. It seemed unfathomable that these basic needs would be unmet for a pregnant woman in a thriving city like Columbus. When we had those initial planning discussions, we didn't yet fully grasp that, central to the threats to better birth outcomes, were the social determinants of health — obstacles including lack of stable housing, food shortages, crime, woefully low incomes and lack of transportation. Frankly, we had no idea the degree of stress under which the moms we were to serve lived every day.

But with our first Moms2B mom, we began to see with clarity what they — and what we — were up against.

Evictions and homelessness proved to be one of the most common, harmful and difficult-to-solve social determinants women and their children faced. That remains true today. In my notes from December 2010, I wrote:

> *Ed Roberts, U.S. Senator Sherrod Brown's central Ohio staff person, visited us and listened intently to our moms. He asked B.T. if there was anything the government could do for her. She said, "No, I'm fine but I wish there was more housing for people. We have a nice CPO house. (Community Properties of Ohio manages public housing in Weinland Park.) But our friends are homeless. We can't have them stay with us because there's not enough room (and they would be evicted by CPO.) We got into our house because we became homeless and went to the family shelter."*
> *As her story unfolded, we heard they had lived with B.T.'s grandmother until her home went into foreclosure and they were all homeless. Then they moved in with her mother-in-law, who suddenly left them, taking all the appliances, leaving them without heat, and a baby in the neonatal intensive care unit. When they couldn't pay the rent or utilities, they went to the shelter. Within two weeks the shelter placed them in their nice federally subsidized CPO house in Weinland Park.*

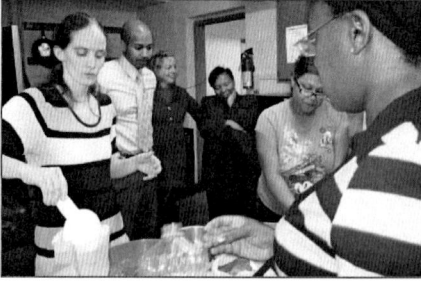

Jen, an OSU Extension teacher, gives instruction in the Grace Missionary Baptist Church kitchen while Ed Roberts from Sen. Sherrod Brown's office and others look on.

As the next decade unfolded, we would work with the homeless shelter board, homeless families support services and housing experts to find more affordable, safe, stable homes for our families. We would learn how the lack of a permanent address caused women to miss notices to re-verify their income to qualify for benefits, how they received sanctions that stopped their health insurance or supplemental income they needed. Without a home, they missed job opportunities. Their older children missed school, changed schools, or failed to enroll in school at all. When they delivered their new babies, those babies lacked a safe sleep environment — somewhere they could consistently sleep alone on their backs and in a crib, free of hazards.

In short, we learned quickly in the early days of Moms2B that we missed the mark with our plans. We needed first to address our moms' most basic needs, and cooking—the cornerstone of our original plan— wasn't on that list.

43201 Mom 2 B?

Are you a MOM 2 B?

Is your zip code 43201?

Are you less than 6 months pregnant?

If you answered yes to the above questions, you or someone you know are eligible for the "Weinland Park MOM 2 B" Program.

What is it?
Be part of a research study, which gives moms:
- The chance to talk with doctors and nurses and engage in other valuable services/programs. You'll also have an opportunity to listen to the baby's heartbeat and make new friends.
- Provides cooking classes while sending moms home with groceries to fix meals for their families.

Where is it held and when?
Grace Missionary Baptist Church, 1182 N 6th Street, Columbus, Ohio (across the street from Godman Guild). We meet every Wednesday between the hours of 11:00am-1:00pm, no need to register, you can just come, child care provided.

Why do you need to come?
- We offer moms the support they need to have a healthy baby and pregnancy, good food, friendships, child care and a small gift card for your time.

For additional questions:
- Call Pregnancy Care Connection (614) 227-9866 or
- MOM 2 B Community Coach, at (614) 247-1983.

Weinland Park has one of the highest infant mortality rates in the state of Ohio. At least two babies die in your neighborhood a year. Please come and join us on our journey for healthier babies.

Our first recruitment flyer inviting pregnant women from the Weinland Park Zip code 43201.

6

Small Program, Bigger Needs

Another early lesson was that we'd shortchange our program's ability to make a difference if we limited enrollment to pregnant women with a Weinland Park ZIP code. Although our pilot program was designed to serve a small neighborhood, we knew that approximately 5,000 Black babies were born throughout Columbus each year, and that each one of them faced higher odds of complications and early death. To make a significant change in overall infant mortality rates, we needed to attract thousands of moms at high risk to our program. We believed that if a woman from another at-risk neighborhood found us, there was no question that she deserved to stay. As a research project supported by Nationwide Children's Hospital, we worked with our institutional review board to ensure that we were within bounds, but also prioritizing Moms2B as a community-based, evolving, service-oriented project — its most important role.

Welcoming moms from outside the neighborhood wasn't the only way we quickly learned that flexibility was key to our success. Though our flyer said: "Come if you are less than six months pregnant," women who were seven or even nine months pregnant arrived for our sessions and we knew that pregnant women at all stages could benefit from our food, breastfeeding support and education about a variety of critical areas, including what to expect in labor and delivery, the importance of spacing pregnancies 18-24 months apart and how to keep their infants safe.

All pregnant women could meet other women and benefit from our group lessons. They all needed to hear: "Your pregnancy is valuable, you deserve good support, come in!"

Research or Program?

As Moms2B quickly evolved — and as it became clear to us closest to the day-to-day work that this wasn't going to be a static, classic research protocol, we invited our larger research team to observe a session in the church. It didn't take long for the group to recommend that we move away from thinking of Moms2B as research and toward thinking of it as a program, but a program that wanted and needed to measure its impact in the interest of continually benefiting moms and babies. The research team recommended we use plain language in an information sheet that explained Moms2B, that we would not disclose names and that we would collect information about them to improve our program. This approach — one free of the rigorous constraints of a formal research protocol — set us free to follow the guidance our community provided us, and to seek inventive ways to meet the needs of moms, babies and families to improve maternal health and infant survival.

One Rule

By December 2010, we had one rule. To join Moms2B, you simply had to be pregnant. Race, trimester, ZIP code — none of those mattered anymore. And we had pregnancy tests on hand to confirm a pregnancy if a woman had not yet had an ultrasound or prenatal appointment.

Many more changes were to come.

Baby and Me

Our next big change occurred with the arrival of the first Moms2B baby. Cherica returned with her beautiful newborn two weeks after she was born. Cherica was bursting with excitement, telling us all the details of her labor, her delivery, her first experience breastfeeding. How could we ask her to leave our 10-week program? After more than two months, we knew these moms, we had relationships with them. We wanted to see them through their entire pregnancy, meet their new baby and encourage their breastfeeding journey.

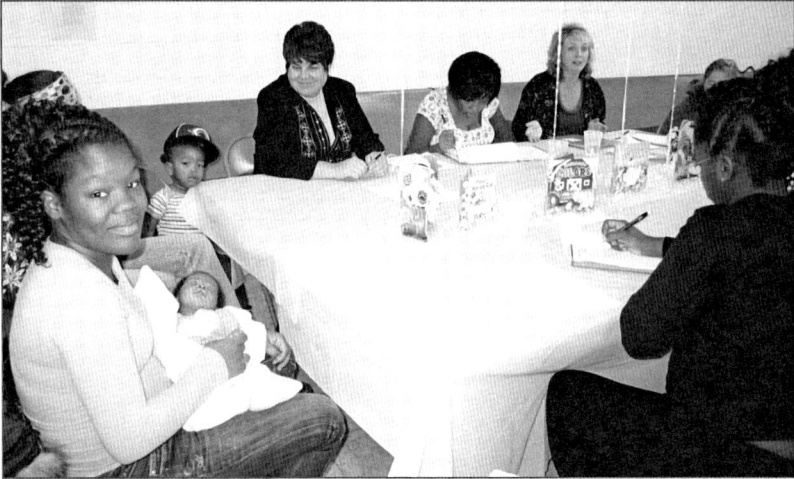

Cherica Dixon with her newborn, the first Moms2B Baby; facing us is Sharon Ryan, a nurse midwife.

We also recognized that ongoing relationships would allow us to help prevent sleep-related deaths — a leading contributor to racial disparities in infant death, claiming two to three times more Black infants than white during their first year of life. We could help obtain Pack 'n Plays and teach the ABCs of safe sleep (alone, on the back, in a crib) and discourage exposure to secondhand smoke.

If the mom stayed in our program, we could encourage her to accept a nurse home visit for herself and her baby and keep her postpartum medical visit. We could educate her on birth control options to safely space her next pregnancy.

A logical step to save babies was to transition from a 10-week cycle to a continuous, open enrollment that ended when the babies reached their first birthdays. Our child development experts started a Baby and Me group for new parents, during which they modeled and taught social interactions that foster attachment and brain growth. They read books, sang, listened to music and toys, practiced tummy time while awake, taught massage, modeled how to quiet babies and showed moms how to exercise their babies' large and small muscles, all to promote healthy development.

We owe it to those first moms — and to our instincts to sometimes listen, rather than lead — that the program unfolded this way.

Lessons Learned that Helped to Form and Sustain the Program:

- We chose a neighborhood with high rates of Black infant deaths and a strong collaborative partnership underway to revitalize the area.
- The pastor and elders of the church welcomed us and shared our vision to help women from the neighborhood have healthier pregnancies.
- Stories we heard from the pregnant women changed our structured plans to teach nutrition and cooking to meet the serious, immediate needs women faced.
- Fortunately, we had the flexibility to change from a research study with a nutrition intervention focus to a program that could meet the social factors impacting maternal and infant health.

2 | Crime and Protection

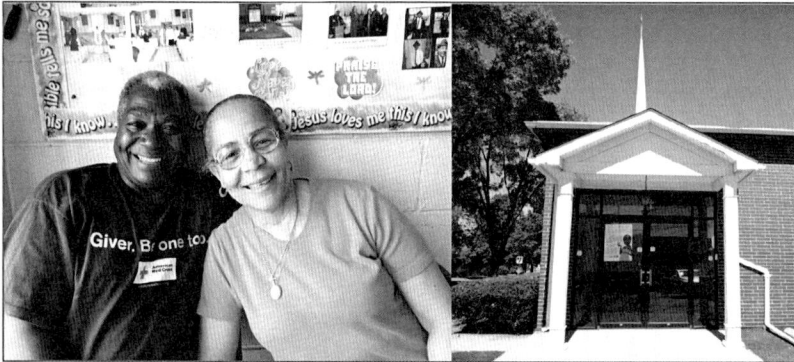

Church custodians Bill and Juanita Bickford and the Grace Missionary Baptist Church in Weinland Park.

A headline in the Dec. 11, 2010, Columbus Dispatch carried news that was a long time coming: "Short North Posse busted." An 18-month probe that targeted the long-active gang on drug, gun and racketeering charges had been fruitful.

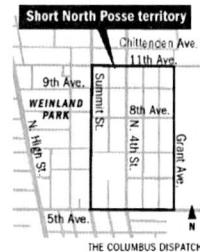

When Moms2B arrived in Weinland Park, crime rates were high. Drug dealers hung outside corner stores known for cheap liquor and a loosie — a single cigarette. People were robbed, shot and murdered with alarming frequency in the streets and alleys. Abandoned, boarded-up homes invited more crime. The neighborhood had a reputation in the community, including among students and faculty at nearby Ohio State, for being unsafe, especially after dark.

That left us with questions about crime's impact on pregnant women, and on new moms and their babies. Did stress and fear cause premature births, low birthweights or infant death?

Before that first Moms2B meeting at the church, we also contemplated seriously whether the safety concerns in the neighborhood made it less than ideal for the women and children we hoped to serve — and for our staff, volunteers, students and community partners.

Before we opened the doors to the church for Moms2B, we visited the police station on the north side of Weinland Park to ask for advice. The chief encouraged us to open during daylight hours and said that if we opened at 11 a.m. as planned we would be safe in Grace Missionary Baptist Church.

Three months after we welcomed our first pregnant women to Moms2B, the headlines in the Columbus Dispatch highlighted the danger in Weinland Park. Nineteen members of the Short North Posse had been arrested, and seven were in custody. Charges included murder, extortion and robbery, arrests that led to the largest federal indictments in Ohio's history. The next day I printed photos and names of the gang members from the newspaper and brought them to our Moms2B session. At least two of our moms recognized the men by their gang names and one mom pointed to a picture and said, "Oh, that's Punch, and he is already in jail for murder." One mom came late, explaining she had been on her phone trying to find bail money for the father of her baby, arrested in the sweep, who begged her to get him released.

One pregnant woman had been at home during a related police raid. Afterwards, she asked "How will this affect my baby? I had to lie flat on my stomach." Physically, both she and her unborn child seemed to be okay. The mom was young and otherwise healthy, and she could feel the baby move and kick. Emotionally, though, she had just experienced severe toxic stress, something she'd likely weathered multiple times in her past. Research has shown that toxic stress causes lifelong invisible scars that can affect a woman's pregnancy, her behavior, her risk taking and the life of her baby.[2]

Afterwards, one mom with connections to the raid donned a wig and dark glasses and darted in and out of Moms2B sessions to let us know she was okay. A man sat outside in a car with the engine running waiting for her. Still, we felt safe in the church. It must have been a sanctuary for our moms too.

One afternoon I drove a young woman home to an adjacent neighborhood and learned, as we often did in the car and the kitchen, more about her family and home life. I asked her about the father of her baby. She calmly said "Oh, he lives across the street, and he's a drug dealer because he has another family to support." Then she told me that when he comes to the home where she lives with her mother and father he leaves his gun on the counter to keep the family safe. "He's nice to me and the baby, he buys us things we need and checks on us every day," she told me, seemingly unfazed by his drug dealing. It's possible that it didn't cause her stress, but soon her parents moved her and her new healthy baby out of the neighborhood.

Crime Threatens the Innocent

Crime posed direct and indirect threats to our pregnant and parenting women and continues to be a factor in the program to this day. The summer after the Short North Posse arrests, during a jazz concert outside on the lawn of the Columbus Commons, a promotional video from Columbus Public Health quoted a Moms2B mom saying how much better she felt living in Weinland Park now that there was less gang activity. Unfortunately, a few gang members who were still free attended the concert and heard the clip. The next day, while she was pushing her babies in a stroller down an alley behind her home, one of them fired a gun over her head and called her a snitch.

This mom, who I'll call Tanya, attended Moms2B every week and helped us prepare our Moms2B lunch. That Wednesday she arrived shaken and tearful. When we discovered why she was crying, we felt responsible because we had recommended that she participate in the video. Understandably, she and her husband did not feel safe at home, especially at night, and feared for their babies and older children.

We decided that we could not let her leave that day without a safe place to stay with her family. Our team mobilized a safety plan, locating a motel eight miles away in a safer area. Twinkle and I checked out the motel to meet the manager and make sure it was suitable for the family. It was a hot summer day and we saw children playing in the pool. It seemed perfect. We gave the manager our credit card, told him about a family that would need to stay one or two weeks and asked him to take good care of them until they felt safe enough to return home.

Crime Throughout our Community

We had other encounters with gun violence outside of Weinland Park that directly affected our moms and our team. In 2011 we had opened another Moms2B site on the Near East Side of Columbus where infant death rates were high. We held Tuesday sessions in a small community room of the Mount Vernon Plaza subsidized housing units. Our team had just finished sending moms home after a noontime session when they heard gunfire and saw a man lying still, bleeding in the plaza. Our moms and children ran past the man to their homes. Our four-person team rushed downstairs and locked themselves in the basement. They emerged unscathed but shaken, more aware than ever of the impact of the stress felt by moms and children in neighborhoods where gun violence is common.

A few months later, a daytime shooting occurred near another location on the Far East Side.

Find a Safe Location

After the third shooting, we learned our lesson. We had moved three times for various reasons and needed a secure site where our staff and moms could feel safe and relax, where we could stay long term, and we were welcome. We found the perfect site in our own backyard at Ohio State University Hospital East. Located in a low-resource neighborhood with high infant mortality rates on the Near East Side, the hospital had friendly staff that welcomed us, a security system, a cafeteria, a large meeting room we could open to the community and, if needed, an emergency department. This new, safer location opened the door to hosting Moms2B in the late afternoons and into early evening, increasing the chances that those who worked during the day could attend. The plan worked: Moms2B East soon attracted more than 50 people each week, plus a growing staff and many volunteers, especially pre-medical students from Ohio State.

Crime Marks Neighborhoods with High Infant Death Rates

In our original Weinland Park proposal, just as we had missed the impact of homelessness, we didn't anticipate the impact crime would have on our moms and on our program. The serious crime we saw in Weinland Park is a threat in several other neighborhoods with high rates of premature births and infant deaths, as documented in a study from the Infant Mortality Research Partnership led by Dr. Steven Gabbe. And we know that historic and ongoing structural racism has driven a disproportionate number of Black and Brown families to live in areas with high rates of poverty, unemployment, abandoned homes and crime — areas where pregnancies too often end prematurely, where babies are often born far too small and fragile, where babies are significantly less likely to live to their first birthdays.

Measure the Impact

Despite the prevalence of crime and other stressors they faced, the moms in the program largely brought with them a spirit of resilience and good nature. "Could any of us tolerate the conditions our moms face and live in and still keep smiling?" Sherry Sheritan, a Columbus Public Health home visiting nurse beloved by many moms remarked to me one day.

To measure the impact of the risks associated with the social determinants of health including poverty, homelessness and lack of safety, we used standardized questionnaires to screen for depression, prenatal stressors or hassles, food insecurity, housing insecurity and adverse childhood events, or ACEs, a category of early life experiences known to cause harm into adulthood. [2]

From these measures we learned how crime, feeling overloaded, work, moving, bills, lack of transportation, the pregnancy itself and finding shelter and food *all* impacted our pregnant women. Every stressful hassle affected at least 15% of women and over 50% said bills, feeling overloaded, transportation and the pregnancy itself caused them immediate stress. Almost one-third of women (30%) screened positive for depression during their pregnancies, 78% had marginal to very low food security and 25% did not have a stable home.

The Life Course Model Explains Black-white Disparities

In the life course model proposed by obstetrician Dr. Michael Lu and pediatrician Dr. Neil Halfon, Black women often begin their lives disadvantaged by being low birthweight, premature or both. [3] If they were raised in a neighborhood with high crime with too many toxic stressors and too few protective factors, such as good food, safe houses and supportive relationships with men, parents and friends, their lives continue with toxic risk factors outweighing protective factors.

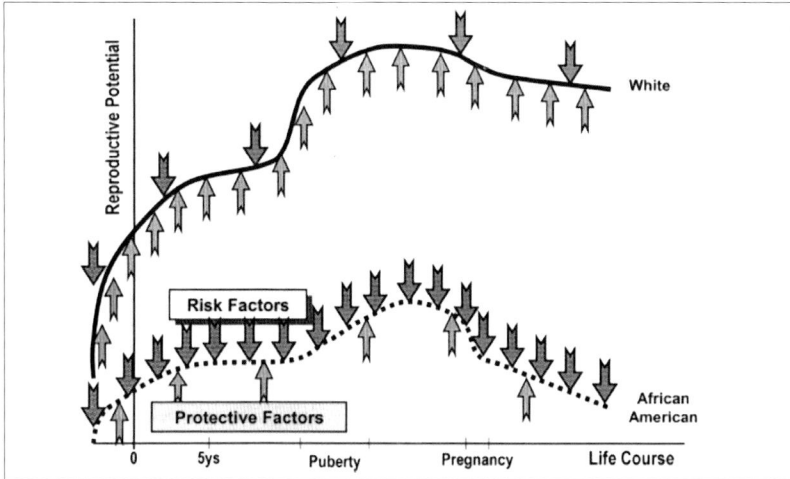

Lu and Halfon, Maternal and Child Health Journal, 2003.

In this model, Black-white disparities begin at birth and continue throughout life. Black women endure many toxic risk factors with fewer protective factors. In contrast, white women grow up with more protective factors and experience fewer risk factors. This environment helps to explain the Black-white disparities in maternal health and infant deaths.

Building Protective Factors

In Moms2B, we soon understood that women needed more protective factors that could buffer the disturbing, persistent risks we identified. Our goal was to soften the material and emotional blows our moms regularly felt. In our recruitment flyer, we used words suggested by our neighborhood community coaches who knew the conditions pregnant women faced.

Our logo, Ms. Apple, invited women to Moms2B because: "We offer moms the support they need to have a healthy baby and pregnancy, good food, friendships and a small gift card." To offer supportive relationships beyond our own model, we connected women to one of the home visiting programs in Columbus. Ohio State medical student Anne Marie Kessler also created Sister-Link for volunteers to support Moms2B women and their newborns after they were home. One mom asked Anne Marie to be her support during her labor and delivery. After the baby came, the father came to visit wearing a T-shirt with the picture of his friend who had just been shot and killed and explained that he missed his baby's delivery because he wanted to attend his friend's funeral.

We felt confident we could build trust and supportive relationships within our program and with our partners. We could break down the barriers to the health care system. We could answer questions related to anxieties about the pregnancy itself.

We needed partners to provide the protective factors of healthy food, improved emotional and mental health and secure housing and had good ideas about how to get there in many cases.

But a larger problem loomed. To make an impact in neighborhoods where residents were at a disadvantage brought on by centuries of racism and experiencing the ongoing threats of crime, poverty, poor transportation, unemployment, abandoned homes and poor schools, business and government leaders needed to step forward. Moms2B could support these women. It could not upend the systemic problems the community faced, and needed support from the public that could only come with widespread acknowledgement that infant deaths and disparities reflected longstanding racism and reflected poorly on all of us as a society.

Lessons Learned:

- Stories reveal individual crises caused by neighborhood crimes that we know causes acute and chronic stress and reflects high infant death rates.
- Pregnant and parenting women from neighborhoods teaming with crime and poverty demonstrate a resilience and spirit in spite of the stress we documented using standardized questionnaires.
- Moms2B builds protective factors for pregnant women to buffer the effects of racism and environmental risks over the lifetime to improve maternal and infant health and with partners, end the Black-white disparities in infant mortality.

3 | Listening and Responding to Basic Needs

"I gained 61 pounds with my first baby, 51 pounds with my son and only 13 pounds with this baby, because I'm motivated to watch my weight and eat right. I'm very happy with the program! It helped me a lot."

–A Weinland Park Moms2B mom

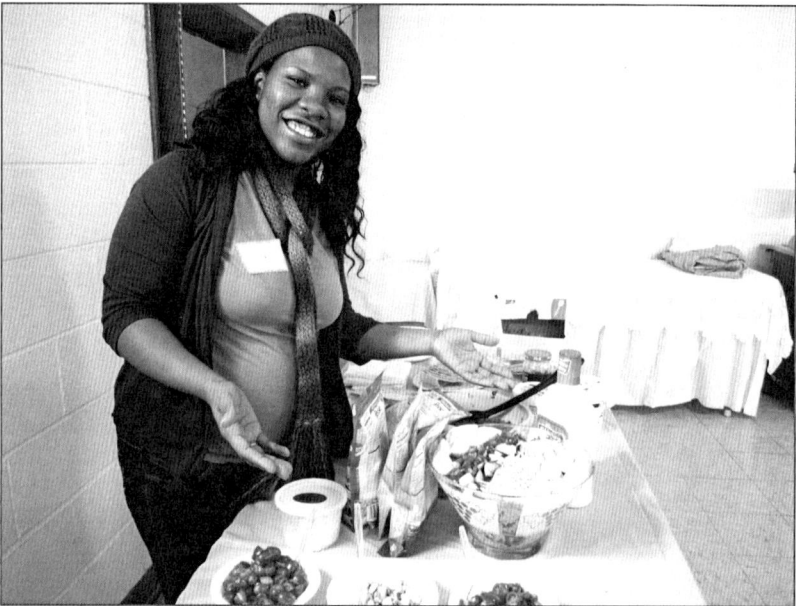

Amber Broadus, a Moms2B mom and AmeriCorps worker, created this colorful salad everyone loved, especially with ranch dressing.

Even as stories of crime, evictions, hunger and toxic family and neighborhood stress were reshaping our priorities, we knew that we didn't want to lose sight of the core of our original proposal: Nutrition. We had quickly learned that moms in our program were often food insecure, and had other basic needs that were going unmet and causing stress on them and their unborn children.

As we sought to reimagine how we would weave this goal into our Moms2B sessions, we asked Ohio State's medical dietetics experts to observe our sessions and help us design a new teaching module for nutrition. Immediately and enthusiastically, they saw the potential to train their students and interns in our unique group model and contribute to our mission. We were equally excited—we knew dietitians could help women access local food pantries and the Women, Infants and Children supplemental food program, teach our groups valuable lessons, provide individualized dietary counseling and promote breastfeeding.

Individualized dietary counseling could also support women choosing to breastfeed and help women with pregnancies complicated by medical conditions including diabetes, anemia, hypertension and other serious risk factors including being obese or underweight.

At the time, only 50% of the women in Weinland Park initiated breastfeeding, and the rate was especially low for Black women compared to white and Latina women. We suspected that a more thorough understanding of the benefits of breastfeeding — and support through challenges — would inspire more women to at least try to breastfeed. We wanted to teach our Moms2B participants how breastfeeding improves their health as well as that of their infant, and that it's cheaper and typically easier once their baby learns how to latch on.

And, based on the diets our pregnant women were describing, most could benefit from individualized dietary advice. I sat with pregnant women every week to review the food and beverages they consumed in the previous 24 hours. Some went long periods without eating or ate too little, while some consumed too many calories, putting them and their babies at increased risk of health problems. Almost everyone ate meals from fast food restaurants and only a few cooked at home. Most of their diets lacked enough calcium, folic acid, iron and vitamin A — all essential building blocks for their own bodies and for their babies. Some women had yet to start their prenatal vitamins. But even with vitamin supplements, our Moms2B moms needed well-balanced diets and healthy food.

Barriers to Nutrition

As a group, more than 80% of Moms2B participants reported that at some point in the previous year they could not afford to eat a healthy meal. Even more distressing, this was often happening in the first couple months of their pregnancies, a critical period when embryos formed organs and grew rapidly. Many were hungry and skipped meals altogether.

What we found in Weinland Park helped explain why too many low-income women and teens give birth to underweight babies, and we knew many of these high-risk situations could be prevented if moms were well-nourished and endured less stress wondering where their next meal would come from. Our moms faced dual stressors: the hunger itself and the ongoing worry about how they would afford food for themselves and their families. Now that they were pregnant, they qualified for the supplemental food program for Women, Infants and Children (WIC). But even women who qualified were sometimes turned away because WIC often faced budget restraints and had to limit enrollment.

In February 2011, I wrote:

"Lelah (name changed) came with her 2-month-old and 18-month-old. At the session Star came up to me and said, 'Do you know Lelah doesn't have any formula for the baby?' I asked why. When she signed up for WIC after the baby was born, they said they were full, and she wasn't on WIC. I asked our Columbus Public Health social worker, Kathy Gooden, 'What can we do?' She said get her down to Public Health, they have a walk-in WIC office. The baby was drinking water in his bottle and was congested. We got Lelah to Columbus Public Health for WIC enrollment. About 6 p.m. I went to the CVS pharmacy and purchased a vaporizer and diapers and took them to her home because her doctor had examined the baby and said he needed a vaporizer that she didn't have. As I opened the vaporizer box...she said, 'I don't have any food Dr. Pat, I've spent my money on formula." She had eggs in her refrigerator, and I told her to scramble them up, they are healthy and filling and we will find food tomorrow.' Twinkle brought her food the next day."

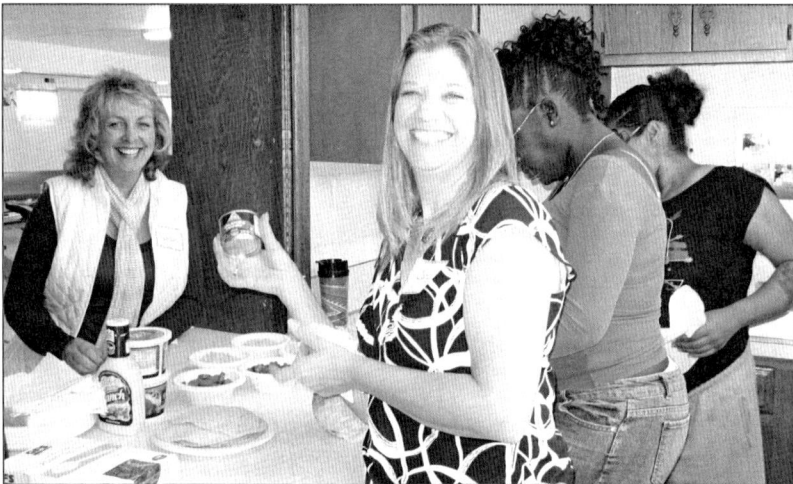

Cooking therapy at Moms2B with Twinkle, Cara Gorman and two of our moms.

Filling the Cupboard

First, we asked the Mid-Ohio Foodbank, (now the Mid-Ohio Food Collective) for help. They volunteered to bring their truck full of fresh fruits, vegetables, milk, eggs and staples to Grace Missionary Baptist Church every month and later to our other sites. This partnership allowed our moms — and elderly neighborhood residents — to choose as much food as they wanted to take home. Because many needed transportation home with the heavy bags, the Red Cross provided it for Weinland Park residents and we arranged for yellow cabs for those who lived elsewhere.

Food banks and food pantries provide one large donation each month coupled with one smaller pickup for emergencies. We toured local food pantries — at Broad Street Presbyterian Church, near downtown Columbus, on the South Side and in Weinland Park — to meet their directors, learn their hours and let them know that when they welcomed our Moms2B moms, they were helping to combat the high infant mortality rate in Columbus. We found the Broad Street Presbyterian Church pantry especially welcoming and well-stocked with food and supplies, often including diapers and baby formula.

In addition to help from the food pantries, our Ohio State dietitians prepared emergency food bags for moms to take home along with leftovers from the lunch meals we cooked during our time together. Six months into Moms2B's inception, as many as 30 people attended each session at Weinland Park. Everyone sat down to healthy, hot meals prepared by volunteers and our team. Communal meals provided a natural time to nurture moms and to learn more about one another as we cooked and ate. Amber Broadus, a Moms2B mom and later AmeriCorps worker, loved to cook and helped us prepare food that acknowledged African American culture. Once, as she cooked greens, she asked me to pick up an ingredient unique to me, a smoked turkey tail. Ed Hoon, a retired Ohio State chef, volunteered to cook our Wednesday lunches and created excellent meals complete with his homemade bread, and menus planned with our dietitian to incorporate food bank items when he could.

Alongside volunteers, dietitians became a mainstay of our teaching program, providing education about how to eat well at home. They mentored students and interns, weighed our moms (an unpopular approach that we eventually discontinued), counseled moms and collected data to better serve and connect women to food resources.

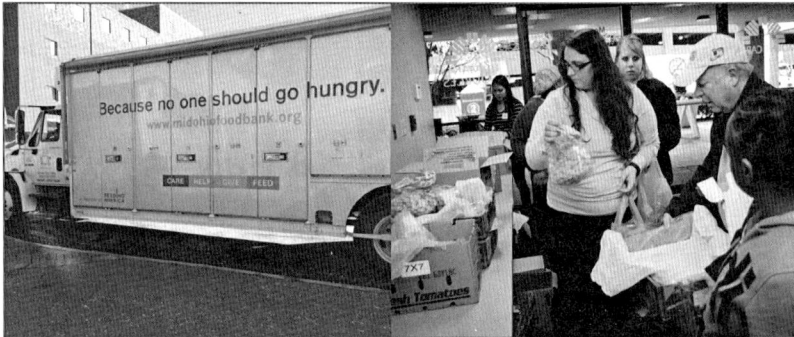

MidOhio Food Collective truck at Moms2B East with fresh produce for our Moms. Sarah Posten, a community health worker, and Volunteer Roby Schottke help fill boxes for moms to take home.

A Weekly Checklist

As part of our ongoing effort to help maintain good nutrition for our moms — and in response to broader recognition that there were core needs that we should continuously check in on — we instituted a weekly checklist that remains to this day. We didn't want to hear stories of moms watering down baby formula or couples spending nights homeless.

We wanted to anticipate these struggles and help find solutions.

Before each woman left, we asked direct questions:
- Do you have enough food for the week?
- Do you have WIC?
- Are you in stable housing?
- Can you pay your utility bills?
- Do you have insurance?
- Do you feel emotionally well?
- Do you want further education or a job?
- Do you have prenatal care?
- Do you have other questions?

This checklist uncovered hidden worries and helped us delve further into the social determinants of health.

Dirty Laundry

The questions we asked opened our eyes to needs we wouldn't have anticipated — matters that might seem small on the surface, but that contribute to stress and erode well-being. One worry that we never considered concerned dirty laundry. Most women lived with their babies and children in housing units with laundry hookups, but many didn't have washers or dryers. They scrambled to do laundry at friends' or relatives' homes or struggled to find the money for a load at the laundromat. And this presented a critical health hazard when bedbugs became a widespread problem in the city.

In response, Katy Calhoun, an Ohio State student in Human Development and Family Science and our first employee, set up a laundry day for Moms2B. Supported by a $5,000 grant from the Columbus Kiwanis, she brought soap and a bag of quarters every week to operate the washers and dryers. To provide transportation, she arranged for the Red Cross van with a volunteer driver to pick up Weinland Park moms and children, along with their bundles of dirty laundry. Volunteers kept the children busy while moms folded their fresh clothes, ready for the week ahead.

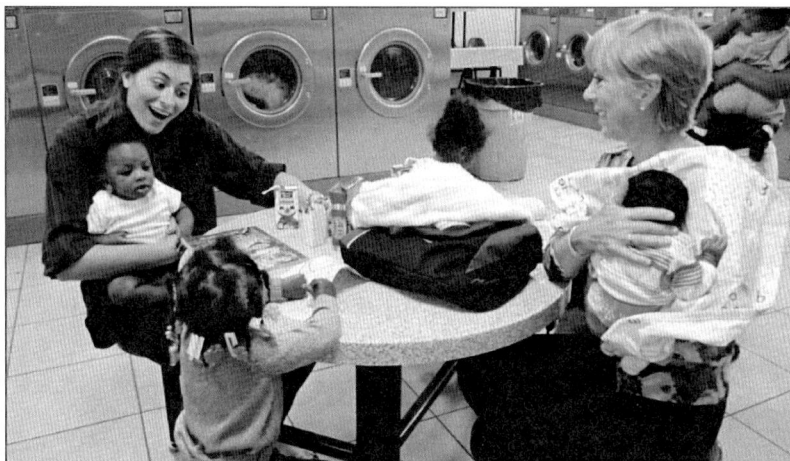

Volunteers Nancy Lockwood, RN (right) and Rachel Welch, an Ohio State pre-medical student at the time, hold babies at Moms2B laundry day in Weinland Park.

The Beginning of Sister Circle

As we worked to better meet the critical, basic needs of the families we served, our sessions began to take a shape that would prove instrumental to their success — to our ability to earn the trust and better understand the challenges these moms faced and to better celebrate their growth and joyful moments in a more deliberate way. The transition from the original OSU Extension cooking course to our own program had led to us setting up "stations" with a nurse and a dietitian to teach lessons and answer individual questions. Soon, we realized we needed more structure and group interaction.

Wanda Dillard, a friend from Ohio State, suggested we start our sessions with a Sister Circle. Sister Circles have a long tradition of providing a forum for women to help women — from simply providing a kind, nonjudgmental ear to brainstorming potential solutions to life's complex problems. Wanda brought a 5-foot polished, carved stick to illustrate how women historically passed the stick to other women in the circle. When the stick reached a woman who needed help, she entered the center and told her story, asking for advice.

We soon adapted a form of Sister Circle to open our sessions. At first everyone stood, until suddenly a pregnant woman fainted. Shocked, I first dialed 991 instead of 911! Fortunately, a physician guest helped revive the mom while we waited for the ambulance to arrive and take her to a nearby emergency room for evaluation and hydration. She quickly recovered and returned next week to find us sitting, in our own Moms2B Sister Circle. We also placed a large container filled with ice water and sliced fruit nearby to encourage pregnant and breastfeeding women to stay hydrated.

Our Sister Circle started with a Moms2B team member introducing herself and sharing a question for the day, often connected to the teaching topic of the day. For example, on a nutrition-focused day we might ask our guests to introduce themselves, share how many weeks pregnant they are or how old their baby is (when appropriate) and "tell us your favorite food." Everyone at a Moms2B session participates — moms, their support people (sometimes dads), visitors, staff and volunteers. After circling the group, teaching topics are covered related to nutrition and stress reduction. (As more dads joined us over time, our circle evolved to be called a Sister-Brother Circle.)

The responses women and their support people gave in answer to the opening question helped us shape our teaching topics and our menus, and provided insight into the moms' emotional health and family dynamics, offering opportunities for support in the moment and in one-on-one conversations with staff later that day.

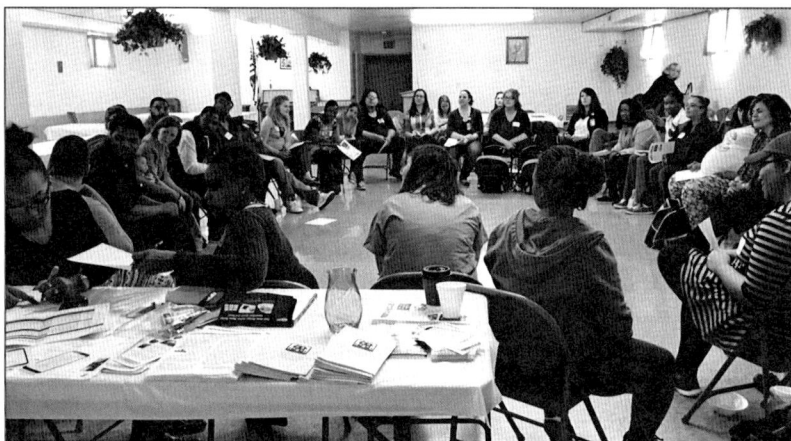

Moms2B Sister Circle full of pregnant and postpartum women, staff, and volunteers at Grace Missionary Baptist Church in Weinland Park.

Our Program Takes Shape

By the second year, we had the basics of our program. We had nutrition lessons, a checklist to alert us to immediate needs and short-term goals, a Sister Circle and a part-time team comprised of an infant mental health specialist, a pediatrician, a dietitian, a family advocate and a midwifery student. Known unmet needs at that point included social workers to help connect moms and families to resources and provide more emotional support, and community partners to better help with material needs. We also had begun to think about how to build a stronger protective network for the moms and babies who were part of Moms2B through a dad-focused support group called Dads2B. Growth, of course, hinged on finding funds to sustain our program.

Lessons Learned

- Poverty robs women of basic material goods and creates stressors that imperil their pregnancy health, especially those complicated by medical conditions.
- Our flexible Moms2B framework allowed us to change our original plans and respond to stories of hunger, to provide food and access to food, building protective factors.
- The trusting relationships, the food and support women found at Moms2B buffered the erosive stresses they often faced in their homes and in their neighborhoods.
- Beyond food and emotional support, meeting the basic needs of shelter, transportation, education, jobs and financial security will come.

4 | Community Partnerships

When I started Moms2B, I was 6 weeks pregnant with my sixth child. I was worried about how the staff would take this information. Upon entering the group session, I was greeted with open arms. No one was there to judge. I also received five-dollar stipends for attending the program. They were helpful with food, gas and diapers."

–A mom living in Weinland Park

The long-term success of Moms2B has come in large part due to a broader community awareness of high infant death rates and a commitment to ensuring access to health care, promoting well-being and eliminating hunger. Our partnerships have been instrumental in meeting the needs of the families we serve.

Kroger

As we grew, and learned more from our moms about their needs, we found more partners and more grant support to keep Moms2B alive. But, from the beginning, Kroger, the Ohio-based grocery chain, and our city health department, Columbus Public Health, were by our side.

When the leadership of Kroger grocery stores in Columbus heard about the opportunity to partner with Moms2B, they readily agreed to join our fight for food security for our families. From the day we stood together at the ribbon cutting in front of Grace Baptist Church in Weinland Park, they have contributed in many

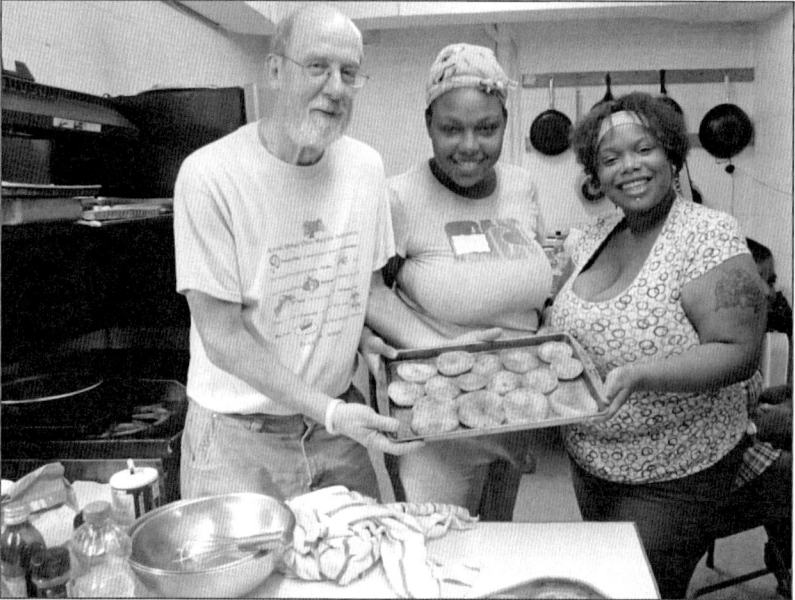

Volunteer Chef Ed Hoon prepares lunch with food provided by Kroger and help from moms Tiffany Bailey and Sharonda Avant.

ways. The week before we opened, we drove to their Columbus office and picked up a stack of gift cards. Each mom received a $5 card for attending a Moms2B session. With larger gift cards, we purchased food for the lunches we cooked every week in the church kitchen. Every year thereafter we met at their Columbus office with our upcoming budget, requesting more each year to meet the needs of the increasing number of women attending. Kroger always agreed to our request, even stepping in with additional support during holidays and emergencies. Though it may seem like a small amount, moms repeatedly told us that they valued the $5 they collected every week. For most of our participants it added up to $50 to $100 before their baby was born and another $50 to $100 in the baby's first year. And moms could accumulate cards to purchase gas, diapers and car seats through a Columbus Public Health car seat program.

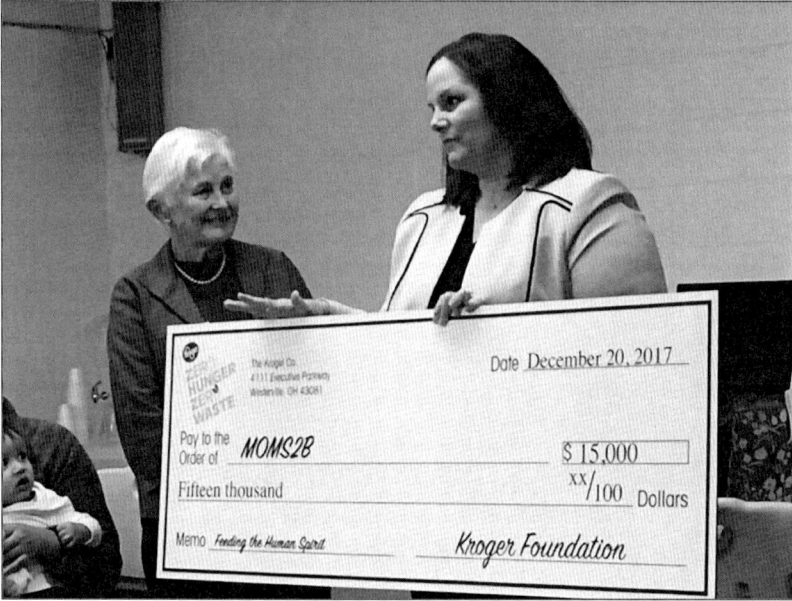
Amy McCormick from Kroger presents me with a check for Moms2B.

Columbus Public Health

Early in our program we relied on experienced Columbus Public Health nurse home visitors and social workers to teach and collaborate on case management. When they saw a mom in need of help, they referred her to Moms2B. When we worried about a mom, they could check in with a home visit during the week. We reinforced each other, and in doing so created a stronger safety net for expectant and new moms.

If the Columbus Public Health team saw a woman at home who had difficulty measuring powdered formula and diluting it properly, they told us and we adapted our teaching style for her. Once, a mom faced eviction because of her poor housekeeping skills and the nurses banded with us to bring her boxes to help her organize, along with house cleaning items.

We believed that our partnership created the ideal model to eliminate disparities in birth outcomes and infant deaths.

However, within two years, their model changed, and we were no longer able to partner on that front. Combining our group teaching model with a nurse or social work home visit remains the best model in my eyes and, fortunately, we saw this later in partnership with Mount Carmel Health.

Columbus Public Health continued to provide many other services aimed at our common mission to improve maternal and infant health. We sent women to their clinics for reproductive health visits, and their successful smoking cessation team helped entire families stop smoking, decreasing second-hand smoke risks that contribute to infant mortality. Columbus Public Health provided car seat safety education and safe sleep ambassador training. Together, we helped women purchase new car seats that were required before they could leave the hospital with their newborns. We helped many women purchase and learn to use a Pack 'n Play for a place for their babies to sleep safely — alone, on their backs in an empty crib.

WIC and Breastfeeding

There was a lady...she talked about breastfeeding, she wouldn't really drill it into you, she more just gave facts and was more down to earth about it. I didn't breastfeed my daughter, but I retained a lot of information that she gave, and I ended up breastfeeding with my future babies because of that...it was more like hey, did you know, like random things about the immune system that you could pass on immunity through your breast milk.

– A Moms2B participant reflecting on the lessons she learned

Central to our mission was making sure that women understood the benefits of breastfeeding and providing support for those who chose to breastfeed their babies. We relied on the U.S. Department of Agriculture's Women, Infants and Children (WIC) supplemental food program for their breastfeeding support, and for their help in combatting food insecurity.

All pregnant women living near the federal poverty line qualify for WIC. After we recognized that 80% of the women in Moms2B were food insecure and that some had yet to sign up for WIC benefits, we formed a close relationship with the director. She sent staff to our sessions to make it easy to enroll our moms for WIC benefits. While they were there, the staff also explained the advantage of breastfeeding, dispelling myths including a common belief that if you breastfeed you can't receive infant formula, or that you lose your WIC benefits. Until we trained our own lactation counselors, WIC peer educators taught these valuable breastfeeding lessons.

That value showed up in community health data. Columbus Public Health epidemiologists measured the impact we and others were making in our Columbus neighborhoods. When they analyzed Weinland Park data for our first Moms2B publication in 2017, they found a steep increase from 50% breastfeeding before Moms2B to 70% afterward. This remained consistent in subsequent studies of Moms2B, leading us to believe that our teaching, and WIC's support, motivated women to breastfeed, improving their infants' health as well as their own. Smoking also decreased from 30% when we started Moms2B to 7% — another critical benefit of our partnerships.

Mental Health

Anxiety and depression unsurprisingly affect more women living in stressful neighborhood environments without adequate financial resources. Most women attending Moms2B have little discretionary income, subsisting on $800-1000 per month, with little increase over the years. Once pregnant, they had additional worries related to their own health and the need to provide for their new baby. And many had histories of prior pregnancy losses and infant deaths and were at increased risk of postpartum depression, a serious and potentially debilitating condition.

In our first year at Moms2B, we realized there was a shortage of providers for pregnancy related mental health care, and community shortages in overall care for mental health. At first, we relied on an organization called Perinatal Outreach and Encouragement for Moms (POEM) that offered peer counseling for perinatal losses and postpartum depression. Later, treatment for depression and anxiety improved as we recruited our own social workers to teach about emotional health and to normalize mental health treatment. Access in the community expanded, and at our own Ohio State Wexner Medical Center's Women's Behavioral Health clinics. Within Moms2B, stigma attached to mental health care also appeared to decrease as women reported good experiences with their therapists and some counselors even came to Moms2B sessions or provided in-home care. We could also refer women to a special POEM program devoted to Black maternal health.

A Big Baby Shower

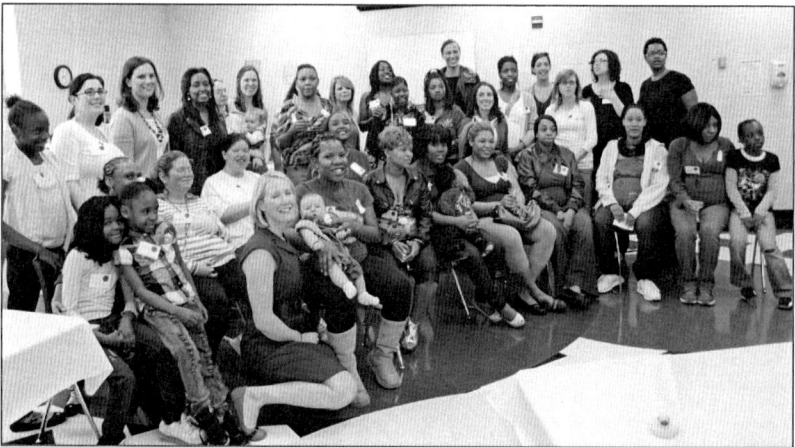

A Big Baby Shower created for Weinland Park Moms2B, 2011.

Early in our first year of Moms2B, Gen Y, a women's professional group from the Young Women's Christian Organization (YWCA) lifted the spirits of our moms when they selected Moms2B for their community project. For months, their group sent a volunteer to Moms2B. They met each woman and planned a spring baby shower with personalized gifts for each mom and baby. More than 50 women, children and friends attended to celebrate moms as they opened their gifts.

New Directions Career Center

"The Moms2B staff helped me overcome barriers to get linked up with the resources I needed. Moms2B enrolled me in a workforce development program with New Directions. After I completed the program, I received a job with Caring for Two." (A Columbus Public Health Home visiting program)

– A Moms2B mom reflecting on the support she received

Most women at Moms2B want a job and those who are already working often aspire to jobs with better wages — the kind of work that ensures they have stable housing, food, transportation and childcare. And many want to further their education and training. Throughout Moms2B, we've encouraged women to follow these dreams. We've helped them recognize and build on their strengths and connected them with training opportunities. Pregnancy, other children, childcare and other barriers often stand in the way between moms and employment. For career counseling, job readiness skills and mentoring, Twinkle, co-director of Moms2B, discovered New Directions, a career counseling and development program that became another valuable partner. They offered our moms a free, intense week-long training for job readiness and career planning. After the course, New Directions' mentorship continued to be available for at least a year.

Female Benevolent Society

The philanthropic group Columbus Female Benevolent Society provided invaluable resources when emergencies came up. When a woman met an obstacle, such as needing to fix her car for $250 in order to drive to work, or to find a refrigerator, a mattress, or a washing machine, the Benevolent Society came through. They invited us repeatedly to an annual lunch with their members so we could tell them more about Moms2B. We explained how their contributions were relieving the stress on pregnant women facing emergencies — an important part of our goal to eliminate and decrease stressors that threaten the health of moms and babies.

Volunteers

From the start, one of Moms2B's most important partnerships has been with our volunteers, who bring energy to our sessions, hold babies, help with meals and help us identify new community resources. We increasingly depended on volunteers as the number of women and children in the program increased. Many volunteers were retired professional women trained in occupational therapy, physical therapy or child development. We felt this weekly two-hour session helped to prepare children for their life ahead. When Columbus City Schools published kindergarten readiness scores showing that Weinland Park 5-year-olds, many having attended Moms2B, were near the top of the list for kindergarten readiness, we hoped that these efforts had contributed.

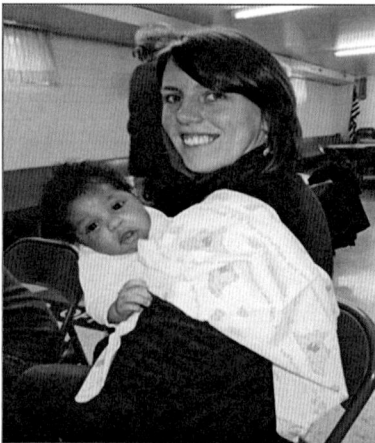

Ann Marie Kessler, a medical student, Ohio State Schweitzer Scholar, and founder of Sister-Link, holds a Moms2B baby. Sister-Link connected moms to a mentor in the community, or a medical student, to help after the baby came home.

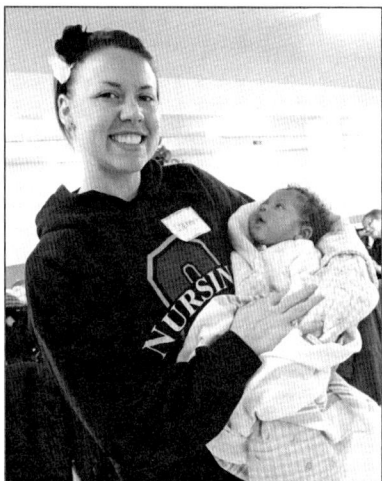
Nursing student volunteer Stephanie
Rittichier with a Moms2B baby.

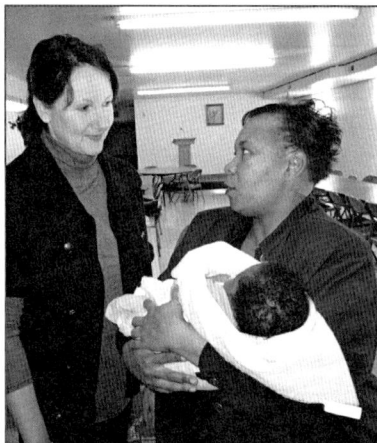
Volunteer Ani Caligiuri speaks with
Susan Colbert, OSU Extension
Director.

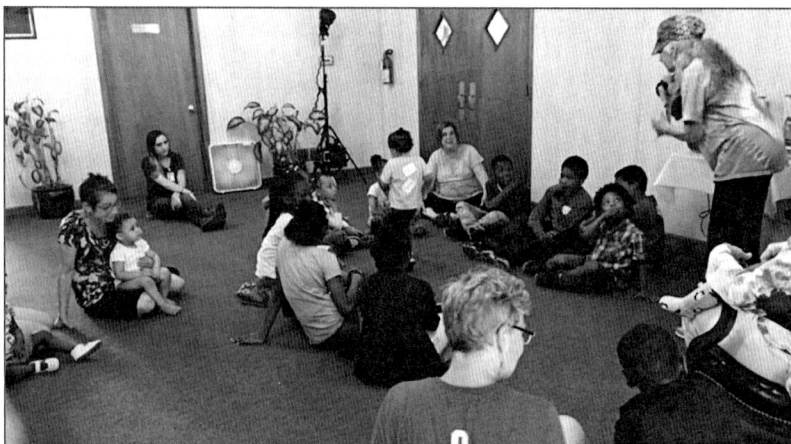
Volunteers hold young children while Mimi Chenfeld, a child development
specialist, engages everyone with her puppet Snowball, her music, stories
and games.

Financial Partners

As the Moms2B program continued to grow, we sought opportunities for funding that would allow us to best meet the needs of the moms we served. The Chase Foundation, as part of their investment in Weinland Park, granted Moms2B $35,000 to hire a part-time social worker and AmeriCorps worker. As we neared the end of our Ohio State Poverty Collaborative grant that propelled our launch, I asked for a donation from the Harding-Evans Foundation based on our common goals of good nutrition and mental health. They awarded $5,500. A volunteer suggested we apply to Temple Israel for a Lurie Micro-Grant, and they added another $5,000 with the understanding it would be used to connect Temple Israel members to Moms2B. We bought yarn to support a Temple Israel knitting group that came weekly to our Moms2B East site, knitting baby caps and blankets, and teaching some of our older children how to knit. The grant was renewed for a second year to support a cooking group that prepared meals in the Temple Israel commercial kitchen. We froze the meals and took them to the homes of our moms after they delivered. These smaller grants were especially valuable when our applications for larger grants were not funded — a reminder that thinking creatively would be instrumental to Moms2B's survival.

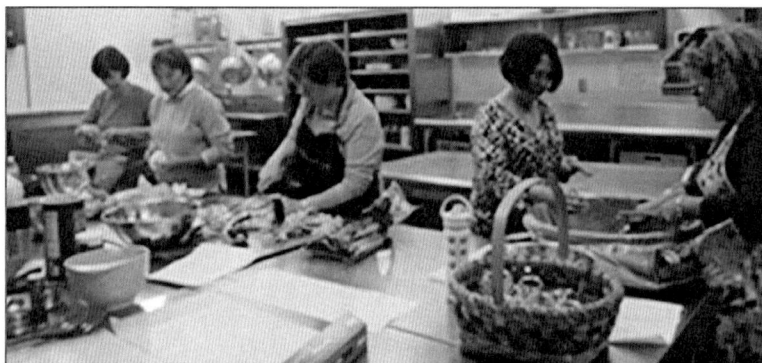

Karen Paneth, a dedicated volunteer, leads a group of Temple Israel members cooking for Moms2B.

A Leader in the Neighborhood

Sometimes our most beneficial partnerships arose from relationships with a single individual in our community. Michael Wilkos was in a leadership position at the Columbus Foundation when we met him. A resident of Weinland Park active in the neighborhood collaborative, he heard about our activities and saw women he knew pushing strollers to Moms2B every Wednesday. The Columbus Foundation was heavily invested in the Weinland Park redevelopment, funding a staff person to support the collaborative and maintain community involvement in the effort. Once our Ohio State grant support ended, Michael helped with a grant to keep Moms2B funded in Weinland Park. Later, when he moved to the United Way of Central Ohio, he continued to support funding through that organization.

Nationwide Children's Hospital

On the other end of the spectrum, major organizations based in our city were also instrumental in our success. As we expanded to the Near East Side of Columbus, Nationwide Children's Hospital continued to pay my part-time salary and agreed to supplement Twinkle's salary. They had explicitly asked us to open Moms2B on the East Side and we were eager, but we needed the dollars to support expansion. My research grant to start Moms2B was managed by the hospital's Research Institute with invaluable advice from Dr. Kelly Kelleher and support from his team. Our partnership with Children's ran deeper.

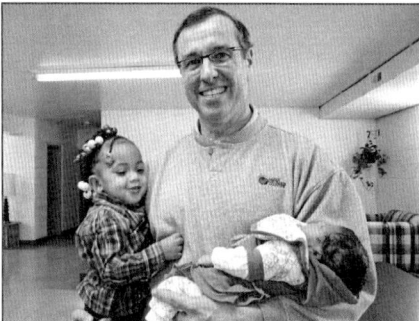

Dr. Kelly Kelleher from Nationwide Children's Hospital holds two Moms2B babies at Grace Baptist Church in 2011.

Their Teen and Pregnant Program referred teens to Moms2B and connected them to the Nurse Family Partnership home visiting program and the newly formed Center for Healthy Families. Both the program and the center shared our goal to promote healthy pregnancies, eliminate disparities and help teens reach their future potential without another closely spaced pregnancy. To assure every pregnant woman received support from one of our programs, we vowed to collaborate and not duplicate services in the interest of optimizing and conserving scarce resources.

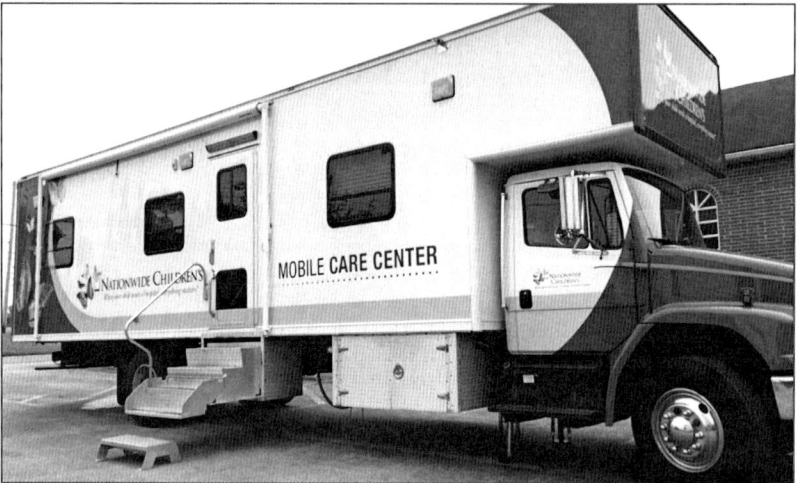

Nationwide Children's Mobile Care Center parked beside Moms2B in Weinland Park.

Another unexpected partnership with Nationwide Children's developed after we found a new opportunity to meet a critical need.

I asked one of our moms with a six-month-old who was mildly ill, "He's up to date on his vaccinations isn't he?" She breastfed and came religiously to Moms2B, and I wrongly assumed she would have taken her little guy to Nationwide Children's for his vaccinations. I was shocked when she shared that her baby hadn't had his shots, and quickly learned that transportation and time were both obstacles.

Transportation, even to a hospital just a few miles away from Weinland Park, remained a barrier for many moms. Public buses would require two or three transfers—inconvenient for anyone, and a true struggle for a mom trying to move across town with a baby and other children in tow. Medicaid managed care organizations contracted with the state to provide transportation to medical appointments, but with a caveat: They needed 48-hour advance notice, and they would arrive within a two-hour window before pickup and within another two-hour window for the trip home. In short, using this service to make it to a medical appointment was near impossible. To make this transportation even less user-friendly, the cars arrived without clear signs that they were for medical transportation or that they had car seats for other children.

So, we thought, "Why not bring Nationwide Children's to Moms2B?" We knew they had two mobile clinics. If they could come to our sites, our moms could walk onto the units with children who needed vaccinations, quick checkups for problems such as skin rashes and stuffy noses, and for other concerns. Within a few months we had a successful long-term partnership with the Children's mobile clinic, ensuring high-quality, easy-access care for the babies we served. Over the years, our Moms2B sites have kept the NCH mobile clinic schedule filled and likely saved lives, vaccinating and triaging infants who needed urgent or emergency care.

Dr. Akua Amponsah

In early 2014, after I gave a Moms2B update to Children's Hospital's large pediatric ambulatory division, Dr. Akua Amponsah asked if she could visit us in Weinland Park. She staffed a Nationwide Children's primary care clinic in the nearby Linden area, another neighborhood known for high crime and infant death rates. Every week, Akua brought her lunch, spoke with our moms, and gained their trust. Most moms lived in the

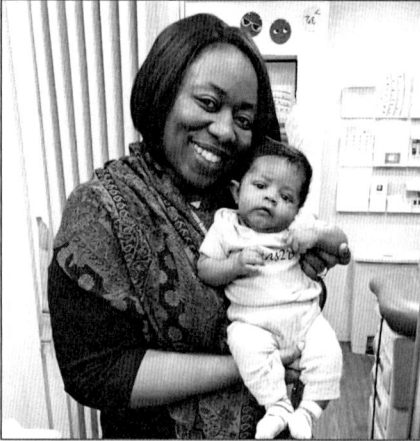

Dr. Akua Amponsah holds a Moms2B baby on the Nationwide Children's Mobile Clinic.

area, and she soon became their pediatrician. When she could, she also staffed the mobile clinic, bringing a trusted, familiar pediatrician to Moms2B every month and helping us meet one of our original goals, to build trust in the medical system.

Public Officials

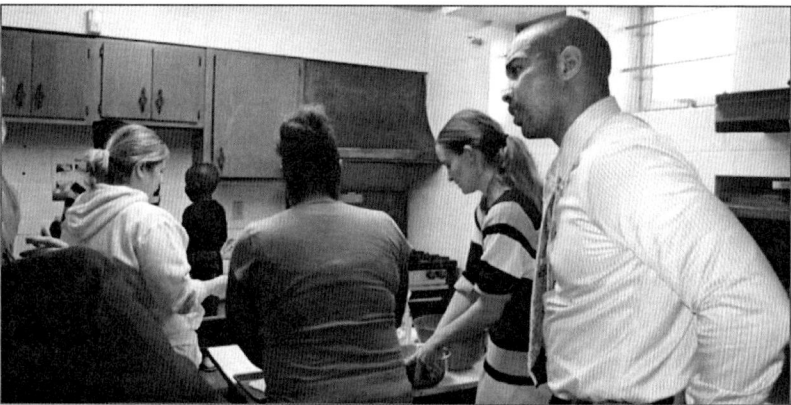

Ed Roberts from Sen. Sherrod Brown's staff visits Moms2B in the Grace Baptist church kitchen in 2011.

After our program prompted a visit by staff from U.S. Sen. Sherrod Brown's office, multiple visits from then Columbus City Council President Andrew Ginther soon followed. Our community work made an impression, and Ginther quickly gathered a citywide task force to study infant mortality and identify solutions. This fact-finding group spent months analyzing the causes of disparities and examining approaches from other cities. They issued detailed recommendations to change the trajectory of disparities, infant deaths and neighborhood decay, creating CelebrateOne, an organization charged with carrying out the task force recommendations.

Our support and relationships with public officials weren't limited to one political party. Because we held sessions in a church, we caught the eye of Governor John Kasich's director of faith-based and community initiatives. Once she heard we were short of funds, she went to the governor, and within days we received fabulous news. The governor had committed $50,000 to Moms2B to support two case managers.

As we expanded to other areas in Columbus, Gov. Kasich's office and First Lady Karen followed through with their support.

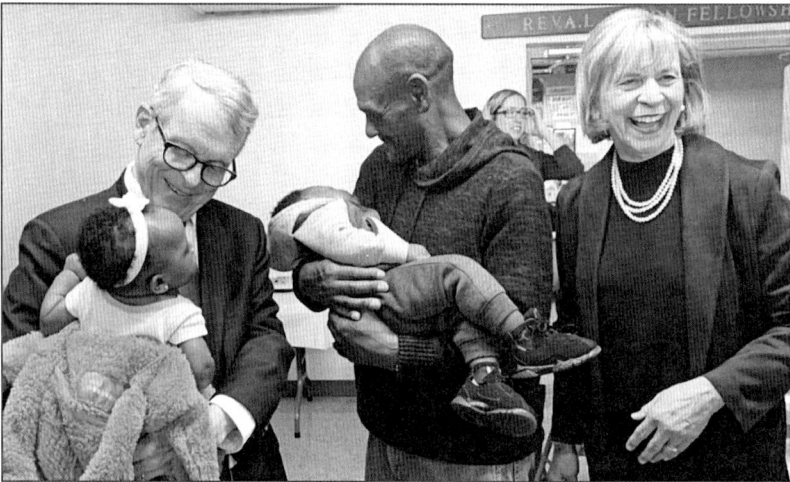

The DeWines visit Moms2B in 2019.

That support continued as Gov. Mike DeWine took office. First Lady Fran DeWine visited Moms2B during the campaign and spoke about it as a model she would like to bring to other Ohio counties. Gov. DeWine designated more funds for Moms2B, and his support has continued for years. On the Wednesday before Thanksgiving in 2019, they even surprised our Moms2B families with an appearance in Weinland Park. I heard several fathers remark, "I can't believe the Governor honored us!" As everyone stood for photos with the Governor and First Lady, one mom said to Gov. DeWine, "I was near suicide, and this program saved my life." With their visit, we ended the year on a high note. Within three months, in March 2020, Moms2B was forced to close in-person sessions and transition to a virtual platform to protect the safety of the community and our team during the COVID-19 pandemic.

Lessons Learned

- It was not well-known, beyond maternal and infant health professionals, that Columbus had a terrible record on infant deaths and disparities.
- Once individuals and organizations learned of the data and our efforts, we found many people generously wanted to help us to save babies.
- Locating in churches and alerting faith-based organizations of our efforts opened doors to more funds, volunteers, and donations.
- Every presentation, media interview, small grant and volunteer played an important immediate role in maintaining Moms2B and many grew into long-term relationships

5 | Ohio State: Our Anchor

On Jan. 24, 2012, in my personal notes, I wrote:

"This is a sobering day. What shall I do to keep funds flowing? Our grant support runs out for a major part of our study. Study? Is it a study? It's a service. It's a service full of heart. But no more funds in our big account after July. Two more months for our AmeriCorps worker and our social worker. How can we limp along, without Tanikka (our community advocate), without money for the Church? Without food?"

Our initial grant came from Ohio State's International Poverty Solutions Collaborative. After the success of our first year, they extended our funding a second year with $48,400. This filled what I called our "big account," set to run out in June 2012, after which Ohio State disbanded the collaborative and our core source of funding. By the end of the year, we faced an empty

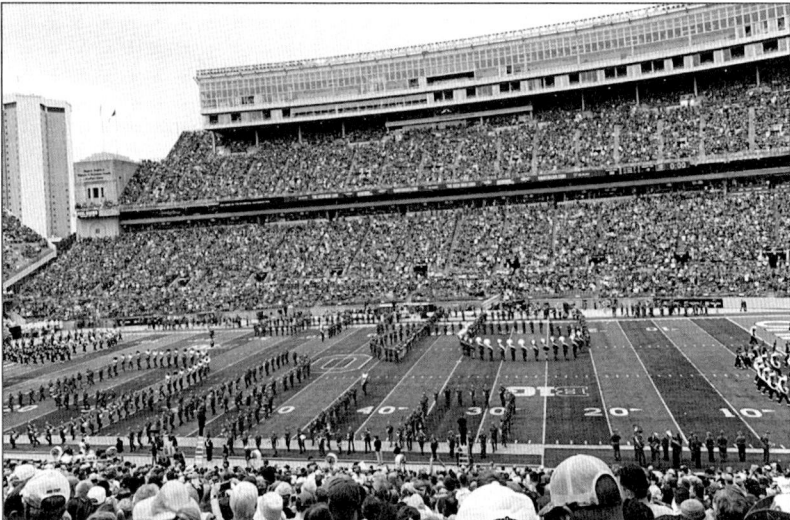

bank account. I was desperate for new funds to keep Moms2B alive, especially because of the successes we were seeing. We had reached many of the Black pregnant women who lived around the Weinland Park neighborhood. We were valued members of the neighborhood collaboration, where we presented data to show the growing numbers of women attending and healthy babies born. We had reached more than 75 pregnant women and 35 babies had been born — all at healthy weights. Sessions averaged about 30 participants each week. We had received good press, with stories in The Columbus Dispatch, Columbus Monthly and the Association of American Medical Colleges (AAMC) Reporter, which featured Moms2B and Ohio Better Birth Outcomes in a story with a national audience. At a March of Dimes prematurity summit in Washington D.C. we presented a poster titled "Moms2B: A group cooking and nutrition program for better birth outcomes." The Ohio News Network filmed us, and the Children's Defense Fund of Ohio profiled us in 2012 as an Outstanding Ohio Practice. In that piece they took note of the sense of safety and community, of the enthusiastic greetings that kicked off our gatherings, and quoted Twinkle, who said, "Our goal is to help moms be successful where they are."

We had momentum. We made a difference in so many lives. And we were determined to stay at both Moms2B Weinland Park and our new location on the Near East Side of Columbus. We had witnessed the impact of poverty, poor or nonexistent housing, lack of food, barriers to health services, stress and violence, smoking, drugs and the racism at the root of disparities in maternal and infant health.

If we could get financial backing, we could maintain this momentum and broaden our program to create training opportunities, jobs and financial security for the women and men who came to Moms2B. We could address the social determinants of health in a holistic way, serving to help reset the trajectory for some of our families. Our partnership with the Ohio State Extension director in Weinland Park demonstrated how we could teach financial literacy, connect men and women to training opportunities and jobs and to stable, safe homes.

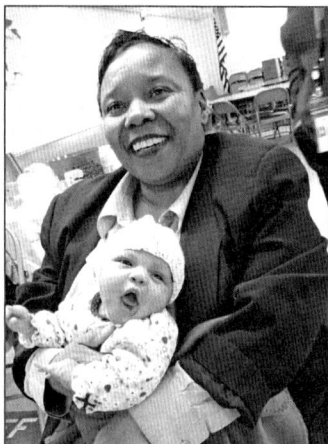

Susan Colbert, OSU Extension Director in Weinland Park, holds a Moms2B baby.

We knew that Ohio State, with their broad range of disciplines, could help Moms2B more comprehensively attack the poverty, racism and social injustice affecting maternal health and causing so many Black infant deaths. It felt natural to ask the university to help us through this financial crisis, in the interest of helping address one of the largest crises facing Columbus and focusing those efforts on neighborhoods so close to the university but so far from its rich resources.

Our Miracle

Soon after I wrote my somber note in early 2012, we heard incredible news from the Ohio State University Wexner Medical Center's government affairs team. Jerry Friedman led the office and knew we had been denied a $500,000 grant request from a foundation, the amount we needed to sustain Moms2B and to grow. Within a month, he announced that the Medical Center received a large award from Ohio Medicaid through its Technical Assistance and Policy Program, known as MedTAPP, which gave us a lifeline of $300,000 and changed our future. These funds were designated to train health professional students to improve access to medical care for Ohioans with Medicaid insurance, and we provided an ideal model for training. More than 95% of our moms qualified for Medicaid, and our model meant that we could place students in the neighborhoods where they'd learn firsthand about how the social determinants of health impacted maternal and infant health.

Receiving the award changed our future and our focus. We could now recruit a permanent staff, enhance our program for moms, add a Dads2B and train health professional students. These new funds gave us a lifeline that led us in a new direction: to seek a permanent home in the Department of Obstetrics and Gynecology in the College of Medicine, a fit that made sense and felt like we were building a program with permanence.

The College of Medicine, Department of Obstetrics and Gynecology

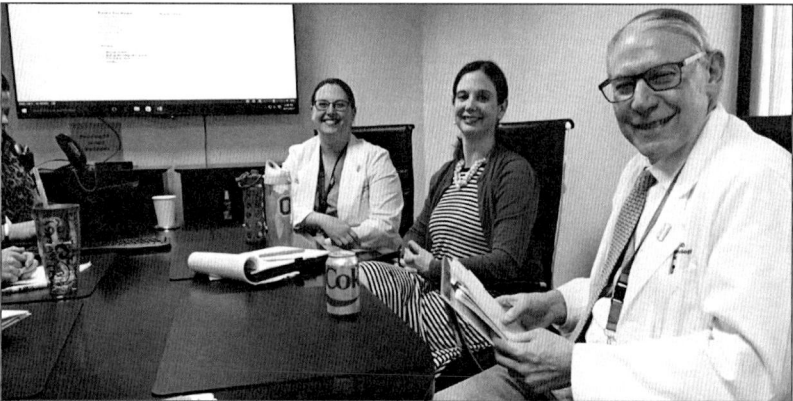

Obstetrician and Moms2B consultant, Rebecca Rudesill MD; Research Director, Courtney Lynch, PhD, and Steven Gabbe, MD, at our research meeting in the Department of Obstetrics and Gynecology conference room.

In the department we found the experienced faculty, clinicians and researchers who helped us form a better connection to the health care system where many of our moms received their clinical care and delivered their babies. The partnership also opened the door to our team attending conferences and staying current on maternal treatment guidelines.

In turn, we could bring stories from Moms2B to the clinical team to help them see the scope of stressors and obstacles these women faced.
For example, just to reach their clinic appointments, I told a group of clinicians:

> *"Pregnant women you see in your clinics are under tremendous stress just to get transportation and arrive on time. Even though their Medicaid managed care provides transportation, it's completely inadequate...One mom carrying triplets would have to be ready two hours before her appointment and could wait up to two hours afterwards for transportation home where she has two other children that need childcare. And transportation passes are limited to 16 per year. One mom with diabetes, without a car, requires twice-a-week monitoring. She has already had one stillborn baby."*

These transportation barriers led us to advocate for changes to Medicaid's statewide transportation system. Eventually, Medicaid's managed care organizations did improve the service.

Expanding Efforts to Hospitals throughout Ohio

Other efforts were underway across the state to tackle the discouraging Black-white disparities in birth outcomes and infant death rates, disparities that made Ohio the state with the highest Black infant mortality rate in the nation, a fact that was not widely known in Columbus and throughout Ohio. Dr. Arthur James, a renowned health equity advocate, and I presented these facts to the Ohio Hospital Association and asked for their help. They promptly introduced five strategies for hospital systems to adopt across Ohio, surmising that if they were fully implemented these strategies would cut infant deaths in half. Now that we were firmly aligned with the Ohio State health care system, we could assist our colleagues to provide:

1. Birth control options to safely space the next pregnancy.
2. Timely prenatal, postpartum and interconception care.
3. Progesterone to reduce preterm births.
4. Breastmilk for every newborn.
5. Safe sleep in the hospital and at home.

Birth Control

Offering safe, preferred birth control methods to women was the most promising way to safely space the next pregnancy (if a woman wanted to become pregnant again) and reduce infant deaths. For the health of mom and baby, 18 to 24 months between delivery and a subsequent pregnancy is widely recognized as ideal. In the population we served, more than half of pregnancies were unplanned and some put the woman's life at risk even though most women expressed a desire to wait until the next pregnancy was safely planned.

At Moms2B we taught women how to develop a reproductive health plan and we heard stories about the obstacles they faced to achieve their goals.

Reproductive Life Plan
Your Body, Your Plan, Your LIFE!

Do you plan to have more children? ☐NO ☐YES
If Yes:
How many children do you want? _____
When do you want to have more children? _____
Are you using birth control now? _____
If NO:
What will you do to prevent becoming pregnant? _____

"They gave me a 'Depo' as they were cutting the cord."

When this mom told us that she was going to miss her next Depo-Provera birth control shot, due every 3 months, because she couldn't get an appointment, I called several clinics to ask if she could walk in for her shot, but no one would take her. She had received prenatal care at an outside clinic, delivered at Ohio State and couldn't get her next shot. This case illustrated the importance of two of the goals presented by the Ohio Hospital Association: good birth control options and postpartum care. A postpartum visit could have prevented this misstep.

We learned that women needed two separate appointments for these services, one to the reproductive health clinic and one to the postpartum clinic. And women with Medicaid faced many barriers to getting long-acting birth control. For instance, some clinics required abstinence for the four weeks before receiving an IUD, or pre-certifications that took weeks for approval. And women who wanted to have a tubal ligation had to have a consent form in place 30 days before their due dates — making this decision one they had to carefully plan and provide documentation to support.

Addressing care

"I'm 23 weeks today, the longest I've carried a pregnancy. Thank you Moms2B, Dr. Iams, Hetty Walker and Tammy Johnson."
- a patient at the Ohio State Prematurity Clinic

Many women come to Moms2B because they have experienced pregnancy losses and need help to have a healthy pregnancy. And beyond their regular support and care at our meetings, we knew it was vital to connect all moms to providers who could support both mother and baby before and after birth, including providing progesterone during pregnancy if indicated.

We also knew that when the day came, it was imperative that moms knew what to expect, and when to head to the hospital. When moms asked questions about kick counts, fetal movements, headaches that could be preeclampsia, labor pains and other concerns, we encouraged them to go to triage in the hospital's labor and delivery unit. There, nurses and doctors would check fetal heart rate, check for premature labor and hospitalize the mom if needed. We repetitively tell moms not to wait for an emergency — to seek reassurance that all is ok, and that approach saved lives.

Breastfeeding

"I never breastfed my other three children. During Moms2B I learned how healthy and stuff it was, and I breastfed my baby until she was a year because of everything I learned in their program."
— a participant in a study conducted by MPH student Misti Crane

Moms2B partnered with nurses and lactation consultants to support our moms when they delivered and initiated breastfeeding. We encouraged moms to put their baby to their breast to taste the "liquid gold" of colostrum that transferred so many antibodies and nutrients to their newborn and to ask for lactation consultants as soon as they delivered. Once moms and babies were home, our lactation counselors and nurses, medical dietitians and physicians continued to help women establish the techniques they needed to successfully breastfeed, ideally until their infants reached their first birthdays.

Safe Sleep

We expected that practicing safe sleep for infants could eliminate more than 10% of infant deaths and reduce infant mortality disparities because twice as many Black babies died in their sleep as white babies, and safe sleep education quickly became a cornerstone of Moms2B. We taught women the ABCs of safe sleep: "Alone, on their back and in a crib". But there were challenges to putting that into practice, as not even all hospitals were reinforcing good approaches when we started.

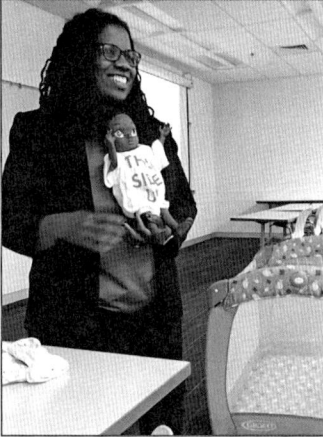

Tanikka Price, our community and family advocate, teaching Safe Sleep with a doll wearing a "This Side Up" onesie and empty Pack 'n Play beside her.

Hospital newborn nurses were asked, through an Ohio Hospital Association quality improvement project, to model safe practices by placing swaddled babies on their backs in their bassinets and reinforcing it with parents in their hospital rooms. Hospitals dressed newborns with "This Side Up" on the front of their onesies.

At Moms2B, we used a portable crib filled with toys, blankets and a baby doll placed face down and then asked women to take out the wrong item and explain why it was dangerous. Still, babies died, and even some of our own well-taught families experienced sleep-related deaths.

Lessons Learned
- Positive publicity and the early success of Moms2B motivated us to secure funding and a stable home for the program.
- Joining the Department of Obstetrics and Gynecology in the Ohio State College of Medicine assured financial stability and access to excellent faculty and staff to teach and improve maternal and infant health.
- Partnering with the health care system helped Moms2B families access medical care and reach their goals to breastfeed, practice safe sleep and obtain birth control.

6 | Ohio State's Many Resources

Beyond the overarching partnership with Ohio State's medical experts and hospital system, relationships with other experts within the university proved integral to deepening our impact and enriching the experience of those who came to Moms2B.

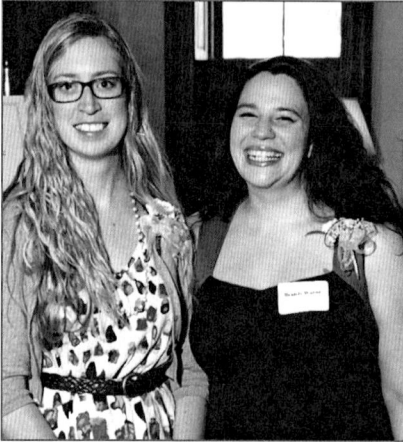

Jamie Sager and Brandy Warne, Moms2B social workers at our 2015 fundraiser.

To Recognize and Respond to Disparities: Social Workers

> *I asked a pregnant mom in her fifth month of pregnancy where she went for prenatal care, and that is when I learned about sanctions that served as barriers to coverage through Medicaid. She couldn't get prenatal care because she had no Medicaid insurance.*

Sanctions occurred when women missed providing their paperwork or missed an appointment required to renew their benefits, often every three months. We turned to Tom Gregoire, dean of Ohio State's College of Social Work, who agreed to partner with Moms2B, both through faculty support and as a training site for students. This led to a lasting relationship.

We hired social workers, and they taught women how to access the services they needed. They developed training modules to teach coping skills to reduce the mental and emotional stress women faced. Soon, students were offered opportunities to learn from our team and contribute to case management to connect moms to essential services and to teach. Women reported that a favorite part of Moms2B was the help they received from our compassionate social workers.

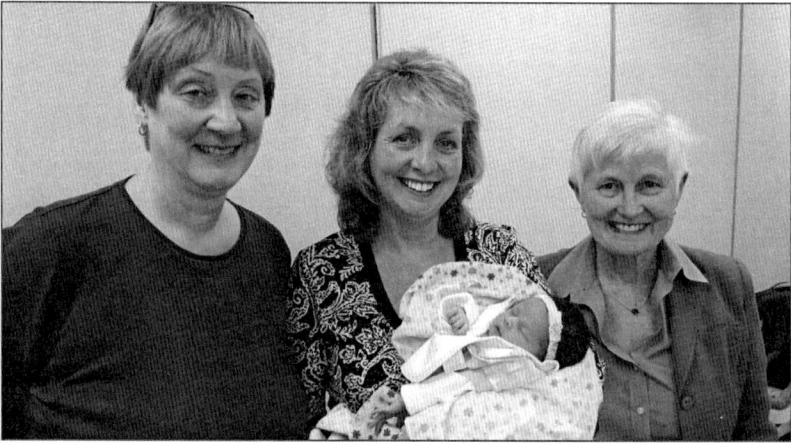

The three founding partners: Nurse Thelma Patrick, Infant Mental Health Specialist Twinkle Schottke and me, Pat Gabbe, a pediatrician.

Nurses Teach Reproductive Health — and Develop Trust

Women worried about their pregnancies, and asked about signs of labor, how to prepare for delivery, anesthesia, backaches, breast changes, sexual relationships, care of the newborn — a multitude of questions that required answers from experts in pregnancy and reproductive health. Nurse Thelma Patrick from Ohio State's College of Nursing brought experience, insight, clinical teaching and research skills and joined us early to help plan Moms2B. Once we opened, she brought invaluable midwifery and nursing students to teach and learn from our moms. This helped build trust in the health care system, especially because most of our moms and dads wanted to deliver a Buckeye baby at the Medical Center. Later, the College of Nursing opened the Total Health and Wellness clinic upstairs from Moms2B in the OSU East Hospital, offering midwives and advanced practice nurses already familiar with Moms2B to welcome our pregnant women into their clinics for prenatal care, family planning and primary care. These nurses are an indispensable and essential part of our program.

A New Stove for the Church

Dr. Virginia Lee, Ohio State's former vice president of Outreach and Engagement, had written her PhD thesis on Black midwives in the South and understood the long history of struggle for pregnant Black women and babies. When she asked how she could help us I told her about our old, broken and unsafe church stove.

Within a few weeks she had purchased and delivered a new safe stove for us. And Outreach and Engagement funded several important grants and awards for the service, scholarship and students we brought into neighborhoods.

An Ideal Public Health Model

Ohio State College of Public Health faculty and students gravitated to our community-based program, and we made several presentations at the college. Dean William Martin and later Dean Amy Fairchild believed, as we did, that maternal and infant health forms the foundation of our society. Their students contributed in many ways. One student constructed our logic model, which explained our methods — especially helpful for grant applications. Students analyzed our data sets and did original research on housing, follow-up interviews with women after they had graduated and supported a mental health intervention to reduce depression and anxiety. The students benefited from their exposure to Moms2B and, in return, we gained their insight and study results.

Women's Behavioral Health

Every week we asked women about their emotional health and well-being. At one session a pregnant woman clearly was suicidal, and the team mobilized a place for her emergency mental health treatment. In this case she refused to go voluntarily, and this resulted in an emergency mandatory hold. The protocol for the ambulance team required them to strap her on a gurney, without regard for her advanced stage of pregnancy. After this incident, we advocated for special treatment for pregnant women and found allies in the Ohio State Department of Psychiatry who changed the protocols for pregnant women throughout the city. Our relationship with women's behavioral health continued to strengthen over the next decade, especially as we developed a strong depression prevention program.

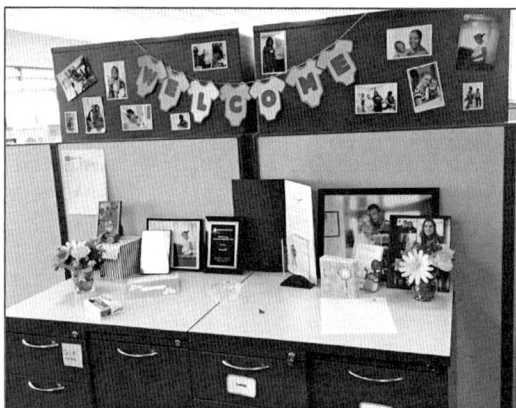

Space for Moms2B

Generous space for our team opened in the Ohio State Health Plan office, allowing us to function as an interdisciplinary team of nurses, dietitians, social workers, community and family advocates, patient navigators, child development specialists and doctors. We could host health professional students, hold constructive case management sessions and store diapers, "welcome to the world" bags, car seats, Pack 'n Plays, and other donations to keep babies healthy.

Moms2B Strategic Plan

Ohio State's CEO and strategic planning office supported our need for careful planning to sustain our program into the future by working with our team to create a plan outlining the opportunities and risks confronting Moms2B and setting a course for our long-term financial stability.

Proof in Numbers: Does Moms2B's Improve Births and Save Babies?

To obtain more funding, we needed data to prove we made a difference. At first, we kept records on paper charts. After almost two years of paper charts, we transferred to an electronic database maintained at Ohio State's Center for Clinical and Translational Science. Our team carried Ohio State laptops to every session, where they entered their notes into a password-protected and encrypted database to assure privacy. This data, along with the partnership of research colleagues at the university, allowed us to begin to answer if and how we were making a difference.

Ohio State University East Hospital, a Safe Place for Moms2B

Moms2B East quickly grew a capacity crowd. More than 50 pregnant and parenting moms, children, dads, visitors, volunteers and our team attended every week from 4:30-6:30 p.m., hours that in many cases allowed the entire family to attend. We had rooms for pregnant and parenting groups and a large hallway nearby where volunteers entertained and played with children. The hospital staff welcomed us and provided plenty of food from the hospital cafeteria.

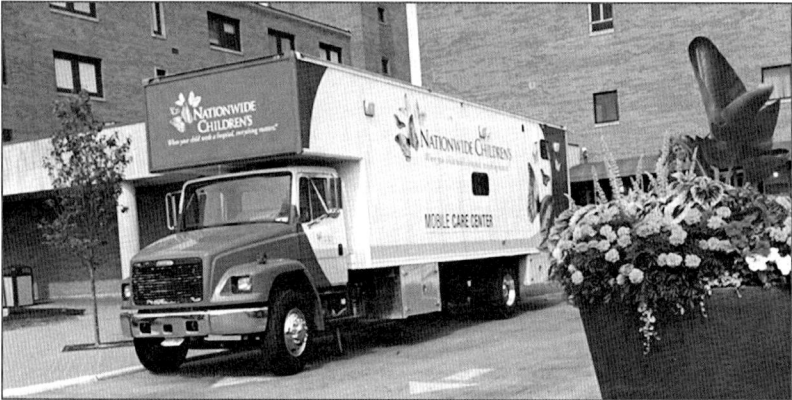

Ohio State University Hospital East hosts Moms2B East weekly and the Nationwide Children's Mobile Clinic monthly.

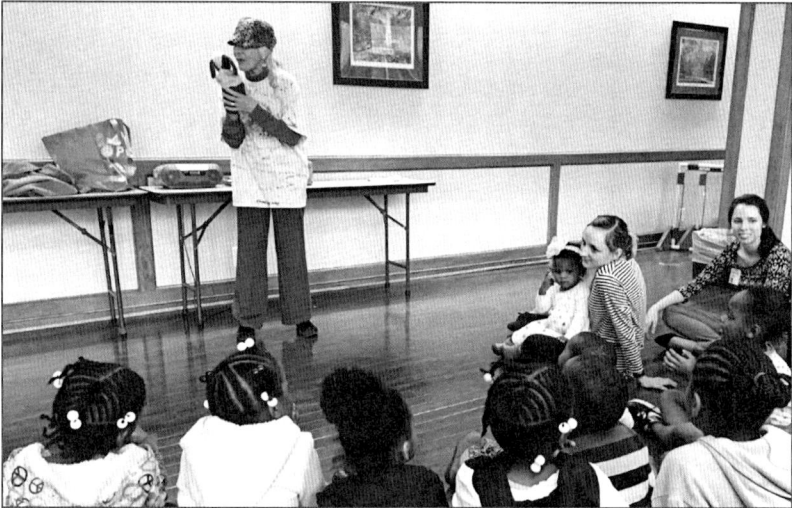

Mimi Chenfield with her puppet Snowball telling a story to children at Moms2B East.

Child development students volunteered, trained and helped immeasurably with our Moms2B child care program at all of our locations. Their home department, the College of Education and Human Ecology had welcomed us in Weinland Park for several years, where they provided valuable space and support in the Schoenbaum Center until we moved to the College of Medicine.

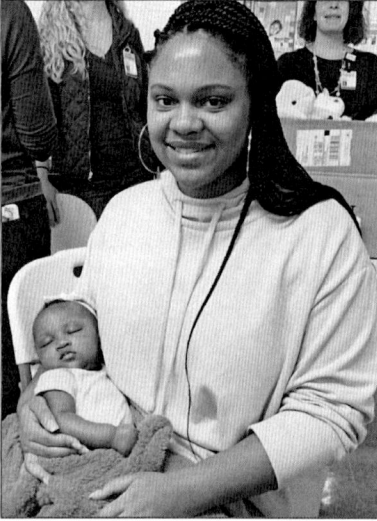

Christian Cook, one of our many child development students. She led our children in their activities and became a long-term, valuable part of our team.

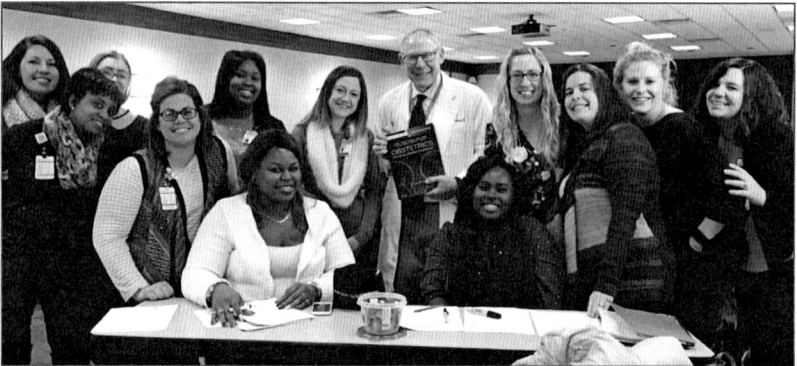

Moms2B Team at OSU East Hospital with Dr. Steve Gabbe, presenting his new edition of Obstetrics: Normal and Problem Pregnancies to our team in 2016.

Chief Executive Officer of The Ohio State University Health System

We returned to Ohio State in 2008 when my husband, Dr. Steven Gabbe, a renowned obstetrician, and dean at the Vanderbilt College of Medicine, became the chief executive officer of the Ohio State University Health System. He was responsible for the delivery of health care, the quality of care, research, education and the business side of the eight Ohio State hospitals, its large medical school and the physician practice plan.

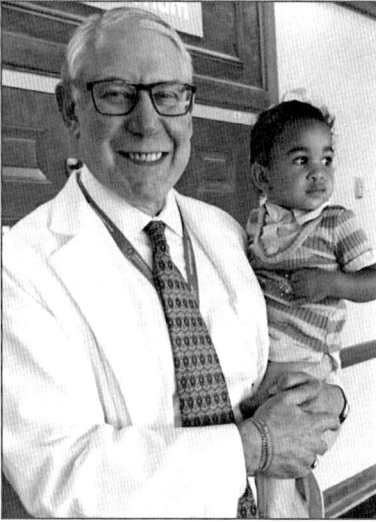

I know his position and his knowledge of the social factors influencing maternal and infant health contributed to the success of Moms2B and helped open many doors for us.

Steve stood behind my efforts to reach into the community and into the homes of pregnant women and those with newborns. He had a long-held passion for the work, having authored a textbook about pregnancy and led research to provide intensive medical care to pregnant Black urban women at risk for a premature birth. That study demonstrated that personalized, state-of-the-art care made no difference in pregnancy outcomes. In fact, women receiving the weekly care with a devoted nurse and physicians had the same number of premature births as those with usual care, prompting Steve and other experts to conclude that more medical care wasn't the solution, and help with other obstacles likely was.

With his position and his belief in our mission, Steve was instrumental in assuring medical center funding for Moms2B, strengthening our future as part of Ohio State.

Lessons Learned

- Ohio State's mission to serve the state, along with its vast array of colleges and financial resources and a top-notch health care delivery system saved Moms2B and became our anchor.
- Combining medical expertise with enthusiastic faculty and students from other Ohio State colleges allowed us to build a holistic program to counter the crushing social determinants of health women faced in their neighborhoods.

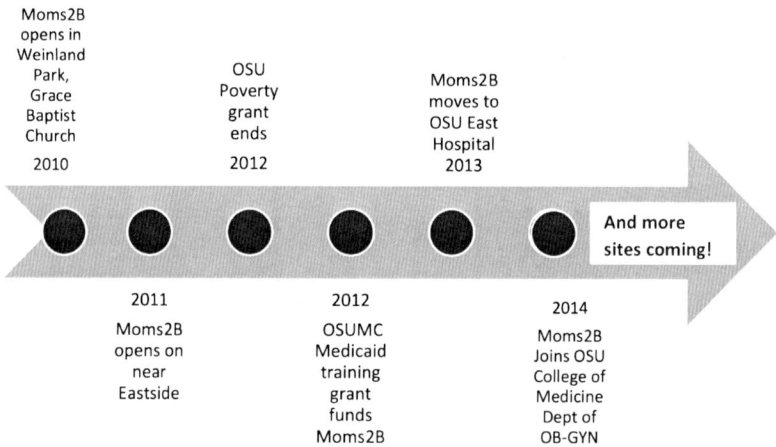

Moms2B opens in Weinland Park, Grace Baptist Church
2010

OSU Poverty grant ends
2012

Moms2B moves to OSU East Hospital
2013

And more sites coming!

2011
Moms2B opens on near Eastside

2012
OSUMC Medicaid training grant funds Moms2B

2014
Moms2B Joins OSU College of Medicine Dept of OB-GYN

7 | A Time of Growth: Mount Carmel Health, Franklinton and the Homeless Population

"A woman just two days postpartum was discharged in the early evening from a hospital, but the hospital was unaware she lived in the homeless shelter and the shelter was unaware she would be discharged. When she arrived, the door was locked, and in desperation, she spent the night on the street with her newborn."

– From my notes in 2018

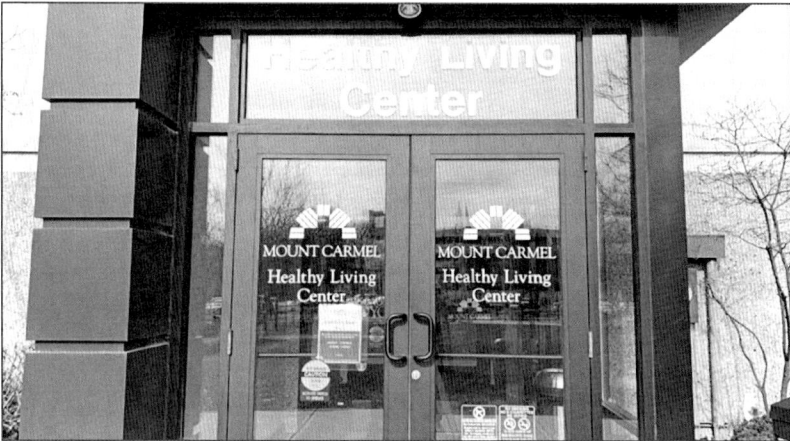

Doors to Mount Carmel's Healthy Living Center, where they host Moms2B every week.

Mount Carmel Health, Serendipity and Moms2B

One evening in 2014, four years after we opened Moms2B, I was introduced to Sister Barbara Hahl from Mount Carmel Health. Sister Barbara, a legendary community advocate, heard me speak about our mission to save babies and reduce the disparities in Columbus. Only a few weeks passed before she asked us to open Moms2B at Mount Carmel West, a hospital serving Franklinton and the Hilltop, neighborhoods just west of Downtown with some of the highest infant mortality rates in Columbus.

We were excited about this possibility. However, we had concerns after we calculated the cost of opening the new site at more than $100,000 a year. We assumed that when we met and presented our budget it would be prohibitive. After we joined Sister Barbara's team and toured Mount Carmel's beautiful new Healthy Living Center — complete with a demonstration kitchen and meeting rooms, and perfect for Moms2B — we met to explain the budget. Without hesitation, they secured financial support from their foundation, a reminder to us that we shouldn't make assumptions about where we might find willing partners, including those willing to make real investments in our community's mothers and babies.

But before we could confirm this promising new partnership, we held a frank discussion about the reproductive health module we taught. We wanted to respect Mount Carmel's Catholic tenets, but we were committed to teaching women about birth control in our group lessons. They agreed with our teaching approach, asking only that we not give individual birth control advice. To our team, that worked out fine because of our practice of referring women and teens to their own physicians for those discussions. Furthermore, many women received their prenatal care at the hospital's clinic, where they were cared for, and their babies were delivered by Ohio State-Mount Carmel OB-GYN residents. This allowed us to not only communicate with the Mount Carmel nurses in the clinics, but also with the resident physicians, who were part of our own department at Ohio State. We did inform women that when their safest birth control plan called for a tubal ligation, it was only possible if they submitted a written request in advance to a Mount Carmel hospital committee. Because many moms we served had serious underlying medical conditions, once they completed their family, a tubal ligation was often the safest method for them.

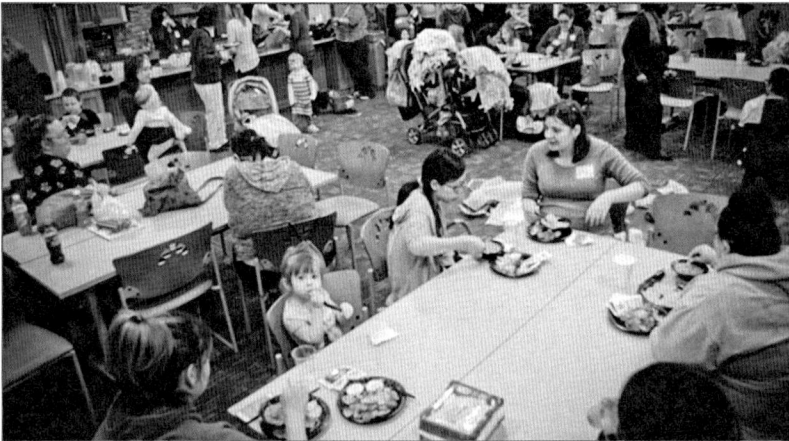

Families eat together after their Moms2B teaching session in Mount Carmel's Healthy Living Center located in the Franklinton area of Columbus.

Serving the Homeless

With the addition of the Mount Carmel site, we began serving more women without stable housing, due in part to the proximity of the nearby Van Buren Center, which serves families experiencing homelessness.

"Black men get locked up; Black women get locked out," Mathew Desmond wrote in his landmark book "Evicted." [4] We found that this was true in Columbus, where most women in shelters were Black. Many had children, and some were pregnant. In some cases, their partners were incarcerated. Without a working partner, women often fell behind on utility and rent payments, especially late in their pregnancies. When they lost their job, they had no maternity benefits, and then moms and their other children were forced to move in with relatives or friends. When those arrangements weren't possible, or fell apart, these women went to the shelter, where they could get help finding a home. The shelter usually paid for the first few months of rent.

With more pregnant women from the homeless shelter attending Moms2B, we explored the conditions there and began to learn more about the challenges homeless pregnant women face. We knew from the stories they shared with us that they were treated no differently because of their pregnancies. They were required to leave after breakfast when the facilities were locked and could return when the doors opened around 5 p.m. for dinner.

During the day, they could search for homes from a list of those owned by landlords who agreed to rent to women from the shelter. This required them to ride buses to hunt for a permanent place to live, ideally somewhere they could settle before the arrival of their newborns. This search often happened with other children along for the ride. Unfortunately, the apartments they were able to rent were often unsafe, with boarded up windows, no appliances, no furniture, and no utilities. If the women grew tired, they could spend the day in the public libraries that always welcomed them and their children, but this was one option amid a sea of challenges, and the moms often struggled during those daytime hours, especially those who had medically complicated pregnancies that required frequent prenatal visits or bed rest.

We approached the Community Shelter Board's director and staff to ask for help. We advocated for changes to help women have healthier pregnancies and the shelter agreed to some, including providing more drinking water to keep women well-hydrated, and supplying healthy snacks for between meals. They also allowed women with serious medical complications to rest in their rooms during the day and added programs to benefit pregnant women and their children.

Despite improvements, challenges for moms without a stable home persisted during my time with Moms2B, and to this day. Even though we had spent years advocating for our moms, in 2018 a mom in our program was discharged late in the day from her delivery hospital and spent a perilous night on the street with her newborn because she could not rouse anyone at the shelter to let her in. We were reassured that the hospital and the shelter would never let this happen again.

Ongoing Threats to Safety

In Franklinton, we also experienced more alarming episodes with our families, teaching us valuable lessons about safety and preparation for the unexpected. Twinkle, Moms2B co-director, pressed charges after one incident in which a father who had become irate during a Moms2B session, and was asked to leave and never return, appeared outside the next week. When Twinkle politely asked him to leave, he pulled a knife and threatened her. Security was called, and the father was taken to jail and later released, claiming he meant no harm. Twinkle appeared at his court hearing and asked for leniency, hoping to keep the family together and that he had learned from the

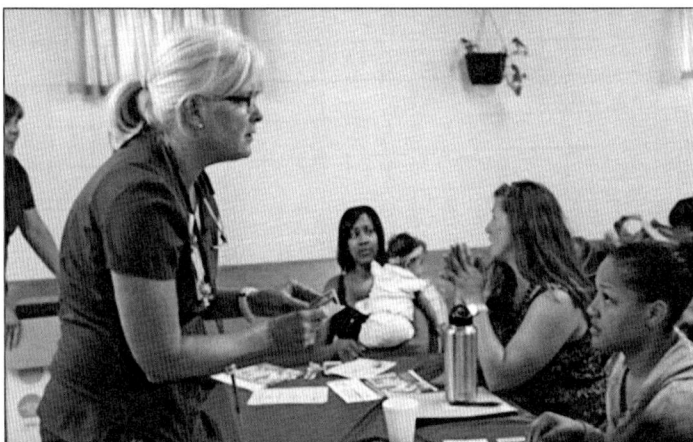

Dawn Elliot, Mount Carmel's Welcome Home nurse meets with Moms2B at Weinland Park. Their nurses attended our sessions in every neighborhood.

experience. He never appeared at Moms2B or threatened her again. He returned to his family, who were living in a tent and would be separated if they went to the shelter.

Building a Bridge into Moms' Homes

Our partnership with Mount Carmel Health eventually extended into the homes of moms, where their Welcome Home nurses made visits that set moms and babies on a healthy path, and undoubtedly saved lives. After one of these nurses would introduce herself during Sister Circle, I would make a point of emphasizing the lifeline that these nurses could be: *"Meet your nurse, she will save your life — be sure to let her in when she knocks on your door."*

The nurses attended Moms2B sites to meet the pregnant women and develop relationships that prepared each woman to expect her nurse to check in after the mom's return home with her baby. In the immediate postpartum period, women benefit greatly from well-trained maternal-infant nurses to assess blood pressure, temperature, healing, bleeding, breastfeeding progress, postpartum depression and the health of the baby. After our partnership, the Mount Carmel nurses began to see all the moms in our program, regardless of whether the mom delivered at a Mount Carmel hospital or elsewhere.

We heard many stories of how their skills improved, and even saved, the lives of moms and babies. At one of our sites a mom who spoke English as a second language had a postpartum elevated blood pressure that needed treatment. Because of challenges presented by language and cultural differences, a Welcome Home nurse accompanied the mom to the hospital to be sure she was evaluated and treated to prevent postpartum preeclampsia, a potentially life-threatening complication.

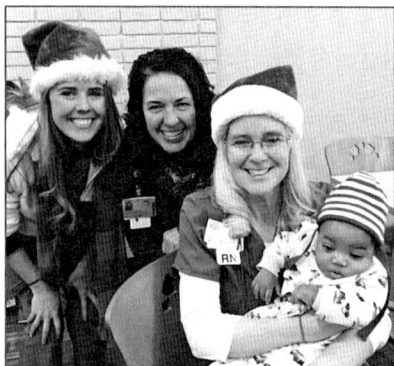

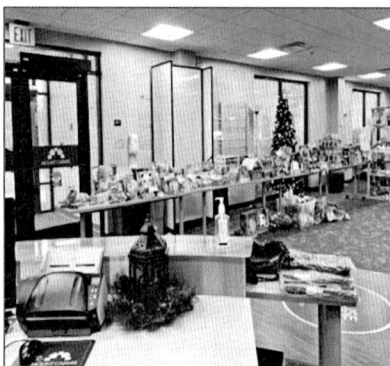

Welcome Home nurses, in Santa hats, and their director, Mary Jo Dickenson in Franklinton with Christmas gifts donated for Moms2B.

And the nurses were also there for the more routine things — weighing babies, taking moms' blood pressure, answering medical questions. The Welcome Home nurses fulfilled our long-standing hope for a continuing partnership between home visitors and Moms2B.

Looking Ahead, Toward the South Side

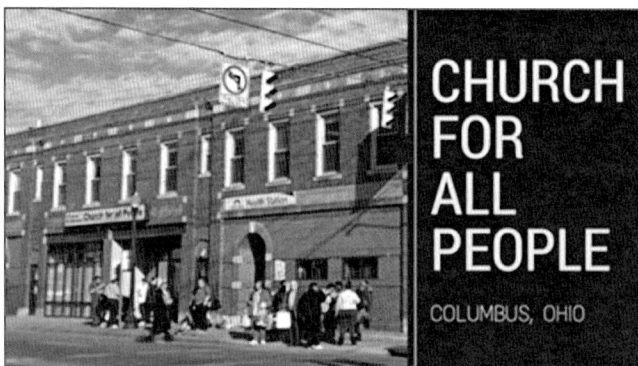

The Church for All People where we eventually found a permanent home for our South Side Moms2B.

As Moms2B in Franklinton began to flourish, our eyes were also on the South Side, where infant mortality rates were high and the potential to partner with other community advocates was ripe. A new Federally Qualified Neighborhood Clinic, now called PrimaryOne, was being built and we had the opportunity to build a demonstration kitchen with meeting space.

At the center's opening event with U.S. Sen. Sherrod Brown, we began recruiting for Moms2B South. In the modern new facilities, we cooked and held Sister Circle in the same room. Down the hallway, a midwife provided prenatal care, and a Columbus Public Health social worker assessed clinical and social histories for women seeking prenatal care. Both the midwife and the social worker had participated at Moms2B in Weinland Park and now we were teammates in this new venture. It seemed like an ideal arrangement, with prenatal clinical care and group pregnancy and parenting education all under one roof. But it didn't take long for us to outgrow the meeting room. We disrupted the staff and clinic flow when an increasing number of moms would arrive with strollers, newborns and children. For that reason, we set our sights up Parsons Avenue to the Church for All People.

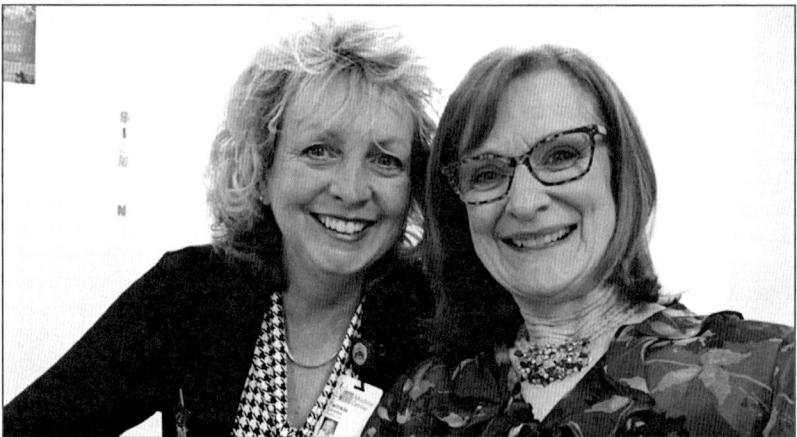

We were invited by our friends, Rev. John Edgar and his wife Sue Wolfe, pictured with Twinkle, to open Moms2B a mile up Parsons Avenue at the Church for All People.

We were invited by our friends, Rev. John Edgar and his wife Sue Wolfe to open Moms2B a mile up Parsons Avenue at the Church for All People. We knew each other from attending community groups fighting homelessness, and the church had a community development arm to serve the people of South Side. They developed affordable housing, provided healthy food and offered other forms of support. An added benefit for us was that they maintained strong relationships with our existing partners, Nationwide Children's Hospital and Mount Carmel Health, which maintained a small clinic next door. The building had space for our meeting rooms and a commercial kitchen where we could prepare meals. Their friendly welcome and our common missions convinced us to open Moms2B South in the Church for All People, where we still hold Monday sessions. Recently, the church stocked a healthy, affordable food market and opened it on Monday afternoons for our moms to shop free of charge. Their efforts, combined with the Mid-Ohio Food Bank (now Collective) truck that added Moms2B South and Franklinton to their monthly delivery routes, have helped relieve hunger and alleviated food insecurity for the families we serve.

Stable, safe housing for pregnant women was then, and remains, one of the most challenging social determinants of health for families who are part of Moms2B, causing severe stress that can impact the health of both mother and baby. Even on the South Side where Reverend Edgar has partnered with a like-minded, successful developer to renovate dilapidated houses and provide low-income housing, women routinely face eviction. In one study supported by a grant that offered 10 pregnant women rent subsidies coupled with intensive case management from the Church for all People, women still struggled. Several of our Moms2B moms qualified for these beautiful homes and were required to pay just $300 per month for a year — long enough, ideally, to allow them to enjoy the early months with their baby before getting back on their feet with a job. But at the end of the year, most of the women had to move out because they were unable to pay full rent, confirming that permanent subsidies were needed. Survey after survey has shown us that about 25% of pregnant women with low incomes are in unstable housing. On any one day, they could find themselves in the shelter, awaiting the birth of their newborn, more likely to deliver a low birthweight or premature infant at risk for severe health complications, or even death.

By the time our Moms2B locations in Franklinton and on the South Side were flourishing, we had a program with strong partnerships to help address the social determinants of health including:

- Racism
- Poverty, financial stress
- Neighborhoods with crime
- Food insecurity and nutrition
- Transportation
- Access to health care
- Anxiety and depression
- Lack of social support
- Smoking and substance abuse
- A safe place for baby to sleep
- Housing insecurity
- Education and jobs

As a result, we expected to see improved infant mortality rates in the years ahead. However, until the housing crisis was thoughtfully addressed with special considerations for pregnant moms and those who'd recently had babies, we knew we would face a major obstacle to lower infant mortality rates overall, and to narrowing the wide gap between Black and white infant mortality rates. This was, and remains, an important reminder that even the strongest supported community programs face limitations caused by systemic issues far outside their control. That said, this realization has positioned infant mortality advocates, including those within Moms2B, as key advocates for safe, affordable housing.

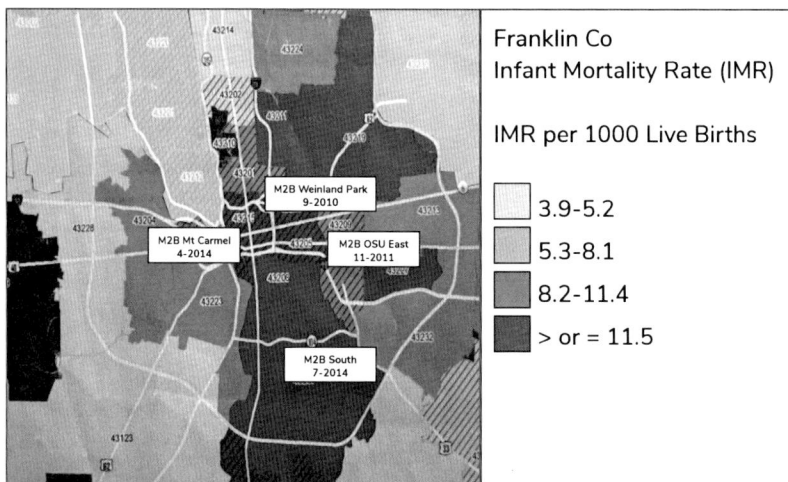

Franklin Co
Infant Mortality Rate (IMR)

IMR per 1000 Live Births

☐ 3.9-5.2
☐ 5.3-8.1
■ 8.2-11.4
■ > or = 11.5

By 2014, there were four weekly Moms2B sessions in areas of Columbus with high Infant Mortality rates (IMR) shown in zip code areas above. Rates ranged from 8.2 per 1000 live births to over 11.5, and in the Hilltop area just west of Mount Carmel, the IMR was 16.8.

Summary and Early Outcomes

In the first four years, we opened four Moms2B sites welcoming more than 500 pregnant women. Each mom attended an average of 10 Moms2B sessions before she delivered, and an average of seven postpartum parenting sessions. Of the 186 births recorded, 12% were born premature — still high, but better than an expected 15%.

Most encouraging, a Columbus Public Health analysis found infant death rates in Weinland Park, our first site, decreased five-fold from almost 15 per 1,000 in the years before Moms2B opened to three per 1,000 four years after Moms2B opened. These results led to a publication in the Maternal and Child Health Journal where we described our new program and reported these improvements.[5]

Now that we had four functioning sites and favorable results from Weinland Park, with the addition of nurse home visits, we wondered if we could expect better birth outcomes and fewer infant deaths throughout our Columbus neighborhoods in the years ahead.

Lessons Learned
- Each neighborhood has a population with a unique culture that requires a program with flexibility.
- Partners with similar missions, to save babies, and a heart to tackle the social determinants of health, last the longest.
- To close the Black-white disparity gap we must assure all pregnant and parenting women have stable, safe, subsidized housing.

8 | City Leadership Inspires CelebrateOne and an Expanded Moms2B

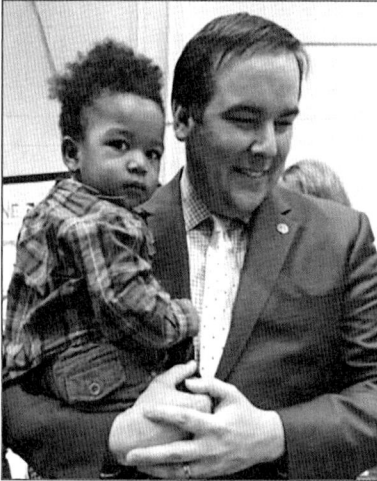

In my notes dated October 2013, I wrote: *"I received a phone call from Andy Ginther, City Council President and he said, 'Dr. Gabbe, I hope you have heard, I am forming an Infant Mortality Task Force, with the hospital CEOs, parents, community leaders, helpful national experts, and I hope you and Dr. Arthur James will be our expert consultants, you will be part of the dialogue, and attend the meetings'."*

Before his call to me in 2013, Andy Ginther had visited Moms2B in the church basement in Weinland Park. He had listened to pregnant and parenting women talk about their health and their neighborhood conditions and how much they appreciated the Moms2B program. At the time of his visit, he was the City Council president, preparing to become mayor of a city that he knew had one of the highest rates of infant deaths among America's large cities — a city where twice as many Black babies died as white babies even though only a quarter of the births were to Black families. Dr. Arthur James, as he mentioned in our phone call, was our mutual friend and an infant mortality expert living in Columbus. Arthur had challenged Andy to change the city's poor record on infant deaths and disparities, and that was one of Andy's reasons for the earlier visit to the church. But he faced an uphill battle. To tackle the underlying causes of the infant death crisis, he needed to convince the public that the problem didn't have one simple explanation. It was not just lack of access to quality medical care, or drug misuse and addiction, or teen pregnancies. These factors certainly contributed, but it was a common misconception that fixing just one of them would solve the infant mortality crisis.

Both Black and white infant survival depended on prosperous neighborhoods and equitable access to health and well-being, in addition to high performing medical systems. To show how Columbus was unlikely to meet the national Healthy People 2020 goal of 6.0 infant deaths per 1000 live births, we compared Columbus with New York City on the graph below, from the March of Dimes.

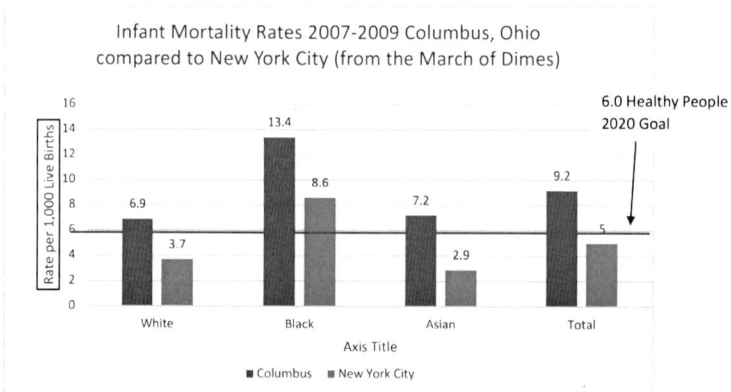

Infant Mortality Rates 2007-2009 Columbus, Ohio compared to New York City (from the March of Dimes)

Category	Columbus	New York City
White	6.9	3.7
Black	13.4	8.6
Asian	7.2	2.9
Total	9.2	5

6.0 Healthy People 2020 Goal

Rate per 1,000 Live Births

Axis Title

Columbus, Ohio has high infant mortality rates for all races and compares poorly to all large U.S. cities, including New York City, shown here. From March of Dimes data accessed 2014.

By 2009, New York City had already surpassed the Healthy People 2020 goal, except for Black infants, a further reminder that even in the best performing cities, Black families suffered disproportionally. Columbus was far from reaching the 2020 goal for all races and had a Black infant mortality rate 56% higher than New York's.

To become a healthy city for babies, especially Black babies, Andy needed private investment in the neighborhoods where most infants died — the kind of investment that would begin to address complex social factors contributing to the problem. And he needed to improve the access to and quality of medical care pregnant women and new moms received.

Soon after our phone call in October 2013, to gain a wide commitment to confront the crisis, he asked 25 leaders from business, health care, city government and the community to form the Greater Columbus Infant Mortality Task Force. He charged the group with studying the causes and developing a strategic plan to change infant death rates and disparities. Donna James, a powerful business leader who herself had been a teen mother, and Mike Fiorile, president of The Dispatch Printing Company, led the task force with First Lady Karen Kasich, wife of then Governor John Kasich, as honorary co-chair. The leaders of all the city's hospital systems were also members.

The task force had impassioned discussions, especially after Ohio State's Kirwan Institute presented research that detailed on maps the social-economic factors threatening residents of neighborhoods where infant death was far too common. The map that follows in this chapter, labeled "Franklin County Infant Deaths 2007-2011" identifies gray areas with few infant deaths contrasted with dark gray spots, within white halos, where 15 infant deaths occur per square mile. These eight dark gray neighborhoods are characterized by poverty, vacant homes, foreclosures, low education levels, juvenile arrests and crimes — creating a milieu of stress and anxiety for families, often Black families, struggling to have healthy babies.

Consider the statistics that burden Black families:
- 32% of Black residents lived in poverty versus 13% of white residents.
- 16% of Black residents were unemployed versus 6.6% of white residents.
- Nearly 14% of Black residents did not have a high school education versus 9% of white residents.
- Black residents accounted for 71% of the homeless population served by the shelter system.

FRANKLIN COUNTY INFANT DEATHS, 2007-2011

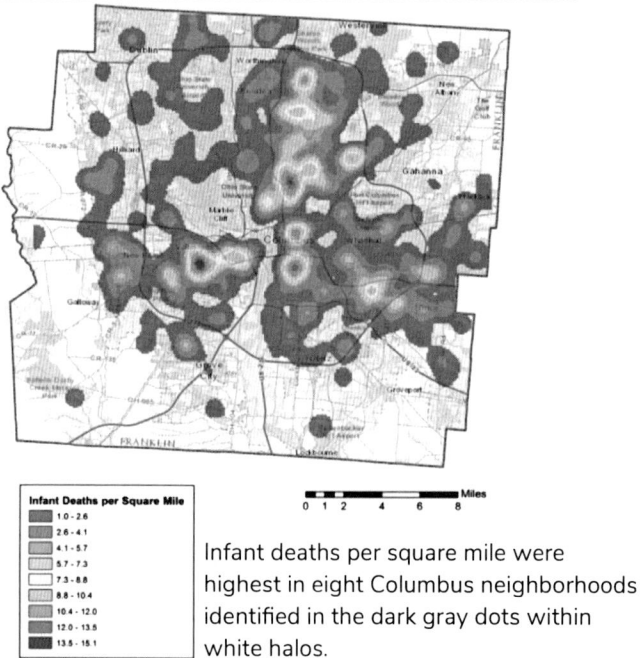

Infant Deaths per Square Mile
- 1.0 - 2.6
- 2.6 - 4.1
- 4.1 - 5.7
- 5.7 - 7.3
- 7.3 - 8.8
- 8.8 - 10.4
- 10.4 - 12.0
- 12.0 - 13.5
- 13.5 - 15.1

Miles
0 1 2   4   6   8

Infant deaths per square mile were highest in eight Columbus neighborhoods identified in the dark gray dots within white halos.

Franklin County families lost 150 infants, on average, each year. Almost half were Black infants and almost half died in the eight under-resourced neighborhoods noted above. These neighborhoods evolved the way they did largely because of racist federal banking standards that drew red lines around areas considered investment risks. Called red-lining, this allowed banks to charge high interest rates in Black neighborhoods and made it difficult for Black business owners to invest in their neighborhoods and for families to own and keep their homes. Redlining, coupled with private real estate covenants that prohibited Black families from living in more desirable neighborhoods, cemented the structural racism that caused sharp divides between neighborhoods. Areas with high per capita income had low infant death rates and those with low per capita income experienced high infant death rates.

It was with this knowledge that the task force completed its recommendations in the summer of 2014 — recommendations based on the mayor's aim of lowering infant mortality by 40% and cutting racial disparities in half by 2020.

The task force issued a strategic plan largely focused on the eight priority neighborhoods:

1. Improve social and economic conditions in neighborhoods.
2. Improve women's health before pregnancy.
3. Improve reproductive health and increase use of long acting reversable contraception (LARC).
4. Improve early entry into prenatal care, especially for Black women.
5. Ensure the highest standards of quality perinatal care.
6. Reduce maternal and household smoking.
7. Promote infant safe sleep and breastfeeding.
8. Create a collective impact and accountability structure to implement the strategic plan. (This objective became CelebrateOne.)

Led by Columbus Public Health and Nationwide Children's Hospital and funded by the city, the health systems and others, CelebrateOne was formed to guide lead entities and partners to implement the plan.

Neighbor-hood Partners	Public Health	Ohio Better Birth Outcomes	Health Systems/ Providers/ Insurers	Social and Human Services	Private Sector, e.g., Employers	Other City/ County

Once formed, CelebrateOne juggled the competing interests of neighborhoods, partners and lead entities to develop interventions that would make an impact at the priority neighborhood level. At Moms2B, we thought we should participate with the partners considering our successful record, relationships with more than 400 pregnant women and their families in four of the eight priority areas, and our intention to look toward expansion in the four priority neighborhoods where we didn't yet have a presence. By the spring of 2016, this milestone opportunity came with an invitation from CelebrateOne to double our sites.

For our organization, this now meant that we had more powerful partners engaged in a more formalized plan for reducing infant deaths and could potentially replicate the successful Weinland Park model of investment in maternal and child health, housing, jobs and education. It meant that we could bring hope for a better future to many more Columbus families.

With CelebrateOne, support we received $600,000 to fund our existing sites, recruit more staff and find churches for four new sites. Four ministers and their congregations — New Salem Baptist in Linden, New Birth Christian in the Southeast, Hillcrest Baptist in the Hilltop area and Epworth United Methodist in the North — opened their doors to Moms2B. By the end of 2017, women and their families could attend one of eight Moms2B sessions available weekly throughout the city.

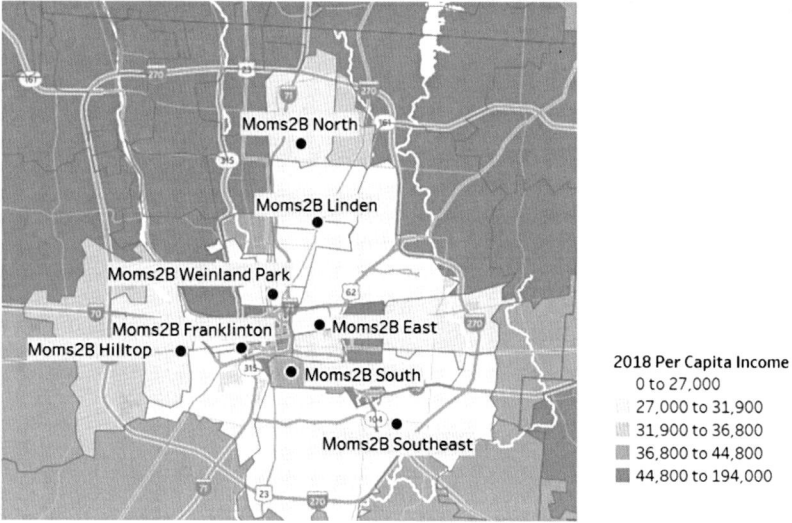

A map of Columbus Ohio shows per capita incomes with superimposed Moms2B sites.

By 2017, Moms2B held weekly sessions in eight Columbus neighborhoods with low per capita incomes and high infant mortality rates. More than half the infant deaths in Columbus occurred in these eight areas.

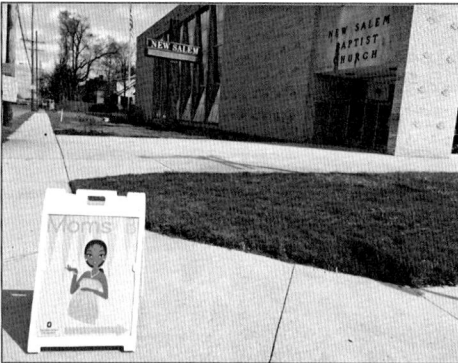

New Salem Baptist Church hosts Moms2B in Linden, on Cleveland Avenue, in an area undergoing revitalization with the city of Columbus and Nationwide Children's Hospital investing resources.

With firmly established outreach into the eight priority neighborhoods, Moms2B attended CelebrateOne monthly community meetings to monitor our collective progress.

We closely followed a scorecard with the numbers of premature births, sleep-related deaths, total infant deaths, the infant death rate in Black families compared to white families, the numbers of cribs distributed and the number of safe sleep ambassadors trained. We monitored whether women accessed prenatal care in their first trimester, whether they continued to smoke during pregnancy and more.

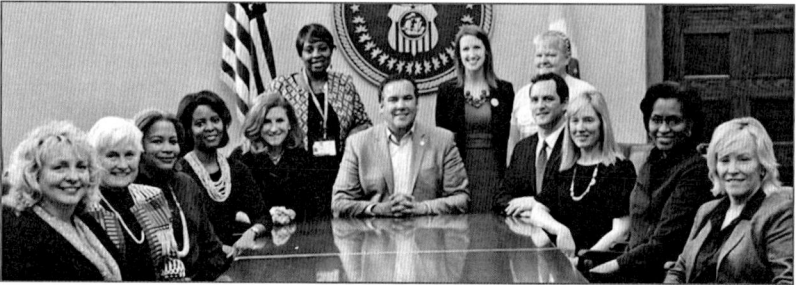

Surrounded by a community group, Mayor Ginther, with members of the Crane family, announces a $500,000 gift from the Crane Family Foundation to fight infant mortality.

Looking back, it's hard to believe we thought it possible that our collaborative, even with all of its planning, teamwork and passion, could reduce infant deaths by 40% and the racial disparities by 50% in just six years, by 2020. Inequities and the social determinants of health run deep and barriers and disparities are persistent.

By the end of 2020 there were 118 infant deaths instead of around 150, and the infant mortality rates improved by 30%. More babies lived. However, more white babies lived in proportion to Black babies, increasing rather than decreasing the disparity in our community.

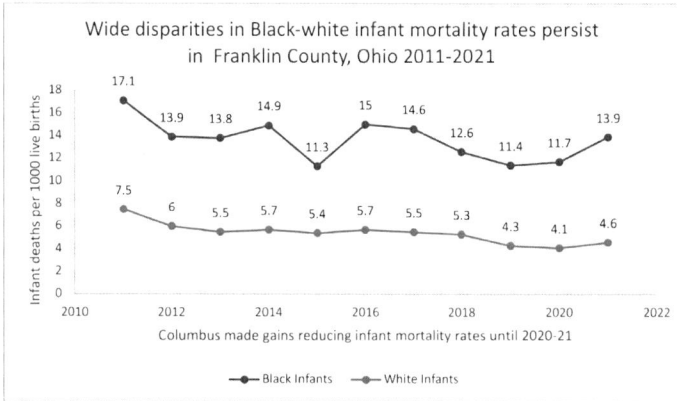

Wide disparities in Black-white infant mortality rates persist in Franklin County, Ohio 2011-2021

Columbus made gains reducing infant mortality rates until 2020-21

Black Infants   White Infants

A graph using Columbus Public Health vital statistics data shows persistent Black-white disparities.

Summary and Lessons Learned

- With strong leadership from Mayor Andy Ginther and in-depth media coverage of the crisis and the work of the task force, the public learned about the real reasons behind the city's high infant death rates.

- Columbus needed collective action from many partners to lead neighborhood revitalization as well as to improve the quality of maternal reproductive health.

- With efforts led by CelebrateOne, Moms2B and other key partners, including local public health efforts, more babies survived.

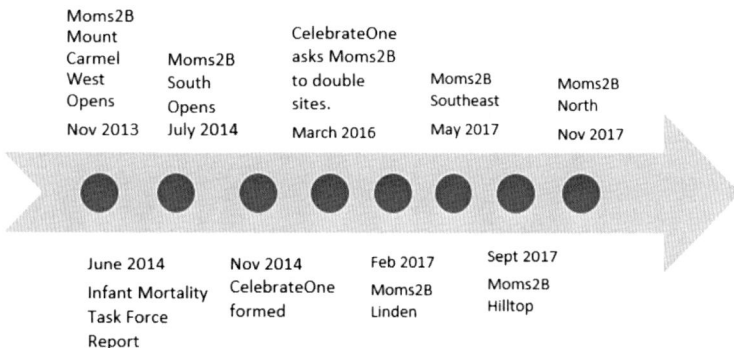

Moms2B Mount Carmel West Opens — Nov 2013

Moms2B South Opens — July 2014

CelebrateOne asks Moms2B to double sites. — March 2016

Moms2B Southeast — May 2017

Moms2B North — Nov 2017

June 2014 — Infant Mortality Task Force Report

Nov 2014 — CelebrateOne formed

Feb 2017 — Moms2B Linden

Sept 2017 — Moms2B Hilltop

85

9 | Dads2B: Meeting the Needs of Dads, Moms and Babies

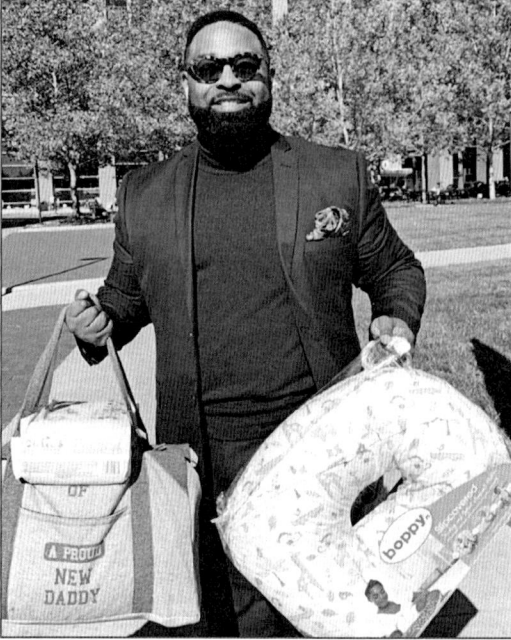

David Fluellen, founder of Dads2B, about to enter the hospital at the Ohio State University with a 'new daddy bag' and a Boppy pillow for a Moms2B family.

Where are the Dads?

Many of the women we met at Moms2B were unmarried, struggled to meet their basic needs and had little support from the fathers of their babies. After women began to trust us, we asked for more details about the fathers. We heard stories about dads who couldn't get jobs because of prison records, those who were good dads but who were spread thin because they had children with other women as well, and those who, new to fatherhood, were overwhelmed and eager to learn more about how to support their partners and babies.

Early in our Moms2B program, a few fathers did come to Moms2B, and we saw how devoted they were to their pregnant wives and partners, how they stayed by them when they had had serious medical complications. We saw fathers take such good care of their children. And yet we heard stories of how they were discounted, or pushed to the side, in situations where they should have been able to be fully engaged. When Joseph, a dad who we met early in Moms2B, went to the hospital with Belinda to deliver, he said *"They acted like I didn't exist. They asked me to 'get out of the way.' They never addressed me as the father of the baby."* Later, we heard Joseph became the sole support and responsible parent for his children. But when his baby was born, he was shown disrespect as everyone focused on the mother.

From my 2010 notes: *"Leandra came to class today, without the baby or her little two-year-old. She told me: "They are with their father; he's a very nice man."* We knew he had just been released from jail and was the father to five other children who had different mothers, but it was important for us and our team to recognize that those factors didn't make him a bad father, or a useless partner to Leandra.

There were also fathers in the picture who caused serious problems. A few examples that I documented in my early notes:

> *"A mother of three, one born when she was 15, then 17, and now 19, told us that the police came a week ago because there was a dispute between the father of the children, herself, and the children. Now she has been put out of her section 8 house. We believe she now lives with her mom, but we cannot reach her."*

> *"I visited one mom in the hospital after she delivered a sweet little girl. The mom was breastfeeding, and alert. She said, 'There was a scene at the hospital, they had to ask Rick (the father of the baby) to leave, he was causing me so much stress, my blood pressure went way up...His adult daughter came into town, that caused a lot of stress. I told him 'This baby is coming, and you won't be there to see your daughter born?' She said he was drinking, that causes a lot of*

stress. I asked her, 'Is he okay with the other three children at home?'
She looked worried for a second, then said 'I need to get home.' A
friend was picking her up at 3 p.m. and it was 3 p.m. This is the
father with the prison record that helped me unload the box of food
last month. A stay-at-home dad."

We routinely screened for domestic violence, knowing that
pregnant women are particularly vulnerable to spousal abuse,
and each week we asked about emotional wellness. If women
reported experiencing violence, and were ready to escape the
situation, our social workers helped them pack their bags,
develop a safety plan, and prepare to go to one of two Columbus
domestic violence shelters.

Dads' Role in Tackling the Infant Mortality Crisis Improves Outcomes

At a minimum, we expected fathers to help with the material
support women and their children needed. But even more
apparent was the moms' need for emotional support from their
babies' fathers. We had to figure out the right way to engage
fathers in a Moms2B program — a way that worked for them,
including those whose history with government, health care and
other organizations may have left them skeptical or distrustful.

Though we weren't certain we knew the best path forward for a
successful Dads2B, we knew the importance of including them.
Children absorb behaviors they see, hear and feel between their
parents and others. The difference between a loving, supportive
home and one in which there is continual turmoil and change
is immense. We wanted fathers and mothers to know how their
relationships directly affected their children's emotional and
physical well-being. Because we started working with families
during pregnancy, we taught that the best time to start modeling the
behavior you want to see in your child is before your child's birth.

But some of the stories we heard from moms — about fathers who were in prison, or recently released, about fathers who had children with multiple moms, about those with contentious relationships with the mom in our program — made us wonder if it was possible to reach as many dads as we hoped to serve. We began to talk to experts outside of our organization and look to the literature.

Studies Reinforce the Role of Fathers

Experts from Ohio's Fatherhood Commission taught us that a father's name on the birth certificate predicted a lower risk of an infant death. Other studies found that children without fathers in their lives were more likely to face abuse and neglect, and experience more behavior problems and school dropouts, as well as have a higher likelihood of becoming involved in crime and spending time in prison. If a father was involved, children had fewer serious accidents, and women experienced less depression and reported more parental happiness. Everything pointed to a need for us to engage fathers.

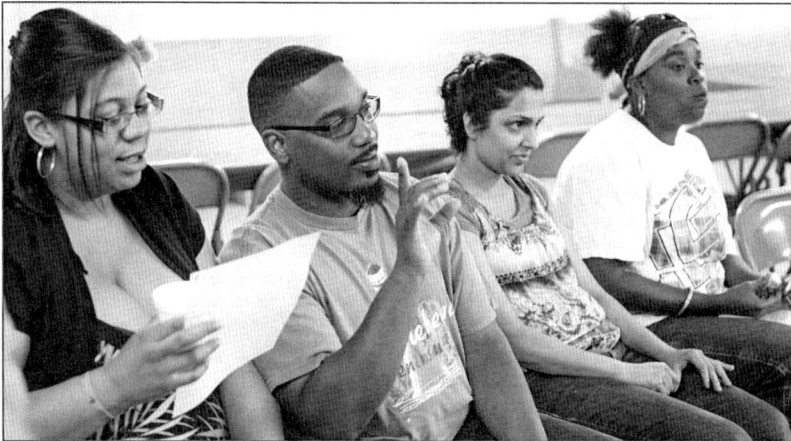

A dad and mother participate in a Moms2B lesson.

Ultimately, we wanted to help fathers understand their importance to the pregnant woman, to their unborn child and to parenting their other children, even if they weren't currently in a relationship with the mom in our program. And this meant we had to seek a new partnership.

Dads2B Becomes Part of the Solution

After several false starts with different fatherhood programs, the Columbus Urban League sent David Fluellen to help us recruit dads and teach a fatherhood curriculum. David had experienced a rough childhood and knew the void young men face growing up in neighborhoods with gangs and without fathers for guidance. By the time we met him, David had a beautiful family, and he loved to teach, calling on his own life story to inspire other men, particularly other young Black men.

By 2015, we had a Dads2B program integrated with Moms2B. David used the Nurturing Father's Program curriculum and brought it to life with his own stories. He helped fathers see how and why they need to create healthy relationships with their partners, to bond with their unborn children and to co-parent their other children.

Dads joined Sister-Brother Circle (renamed to welcome our new attendees) every week, where they introduced themselves and their unborn child and told us about their other children. It was a tremendously important and exciting time for Moms2B that dads were now more formally part of the solution. They heard the same lessons that moms heard on nutrition, breastfeeding and emotional wellness; they joined lessons on safe-sleep, smoking, substance use, reproductive health and birth control. Once a month, David taught the large Moms2B lesson that included mothers and fathers together. Other weeks, after lessons held in

Sister-Brother circle, dads gathered in their own group, where they covered topics including:

- Effective family communication techniques to strengthen father-child and father-mother relationships.
- The secrets for creating safe, loving, stable and nurtured families.
- How to achieve teamwork in family life.
- How to stop fighting and arguing by using proven strategies for conflict resolution and problem solving.
- Positive father-friendly discipline tools for successful child behavior management.

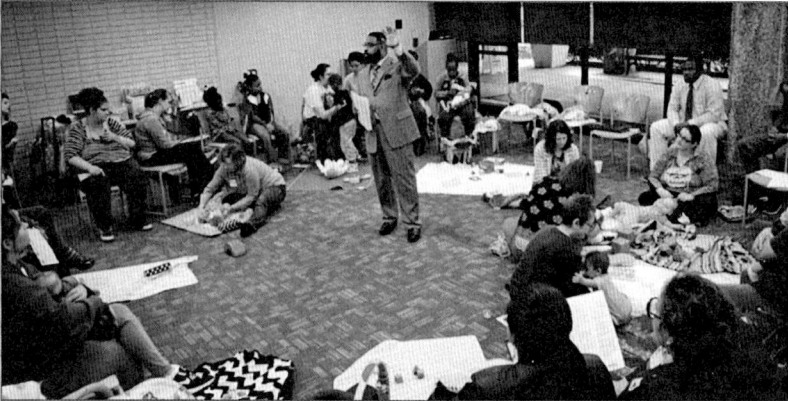

David Fluellen teaches a co-parenting lesson at Moms2B Franklinton.

To coordinate with our Moms2B infant mortality reduction goals, David added these topics to the curriculum:

- Support breastfeeding.
- Attend prenatal clinic visits.
- Learn the signs of early labor.
- Know the social determinants of health and how you can help.
- Stop smoking and exposing baby to secondhand smoke.
- Practice the ABCs — Alone, on their Back, in a Crib for safe sleep and train with Columbus Public Health to become a Safe Sleep Ambassador.
- Safely space the next pregnancy; use birth control.
- Accept nurse home visitors.

With supportive case management, the Dads2B program helped men find jobs, bought work boots or clothes for job interviews and helped with car repairs so that dads could drive to work. They connected dads with food pantries, housing, mental health services and legal aid. They taught the importance of men's health and connected men, many of whom did not have a doctor, to primary care at Ohio State Family Medicine or the Community Care Mobile Coach.

David's presence was always helpful, especially during challenging moments, such as when occasionally a father disrupted a session, or attended a Moms2B session with one woman and had fathered a baby of another woman attending the same session. Together, we tactfully handled all these situations, modeling calm, respectful conflict resolution.

Another area of conflict involved paternity rights and child support payments. Before we had a Dads2B program, a regular mom, usually very quiet, arrived happy one day to let us know that the father of her two children had moved back in with her. However, within a week she returned distraught because he became angry and moved out when he was presented with papers that she had previously filed requiring him to provide child support. With a Dads2B program integrated with Moms2B we hoped to learn how to help families avoid these kinds of unfortunate events that separated families.

Policies that Hurt Parents: the Benefit Cliff

"Kayla was evicted because the father of the babies was in the house, and he was not supposed to be there — he wasn't on the lease."
                                        – a note from my Moms2B journal.

Most of the moms we served lived in housing subsidized by the federal government, and one of the requirements was that, unless the father was on the lease, he was limited to a few overnight stays a month. The catch was that families faced financial disincentives if a father was on the lease. Subsidized housing rents can be as low as $10 per month, depending on monthly income and number of children. To receive housing and other government benefits, families must report any change in income, and they must reapply — usually every three months. If their income increases, even by a dollar, it can mean losing benefits including housing subsidies, food vouchers, Medicaid, childcare subsidies, Head Start and Early Head Start, Temporary Assistance for Needy Families and Women Infant and Children (WIC) supplemental food benefits. Among those who work with families in need this phenomenon is commonly called the benefit cliff, and it's especially hard on contract workers. In our program, it was particularly pronounced for those families where a dad (or mom) made a good income during the summer construction months but had little or no income during the winter. We often heard, "He's at work, but we can't live together because he's not on the lease." This was a disincentive to marry or consistently co-parent, and adversely affected the role of the father in low-income families. These benefits help so many families, but the cliff continues to keep families apart.

Did Dads2B Succeed?

We met one important measure of success: men came and returned. By 2019, after four years of Dads2B, 363 fathers had attended. When surveyed, most fathers indicated that they had attended the program more than five times, with over half reporting that they had attended 10 or more times. Many reported that their parenting and co-parenting abilities improved, and they appreciated a better understanding of their child's development. Most said they received a good balance of support and information.

But we wanted higher attendance. Though new dads were arriving each week, attendance by dads was only about a quarter of attendance by moms. Fathers who worked found they could only attend late afternoon sessions, which boosted attendance at Moms2B East.

Success also meant Dads2B needed to add another staff person, a patient navigator to recruit more dads, connect them with services and maintain the close relationships required for success. Using funds from Medicaid's Patient Care Innovation Awards, we were able to secure support through Ohio State and hire Louis Pollard to assist David.

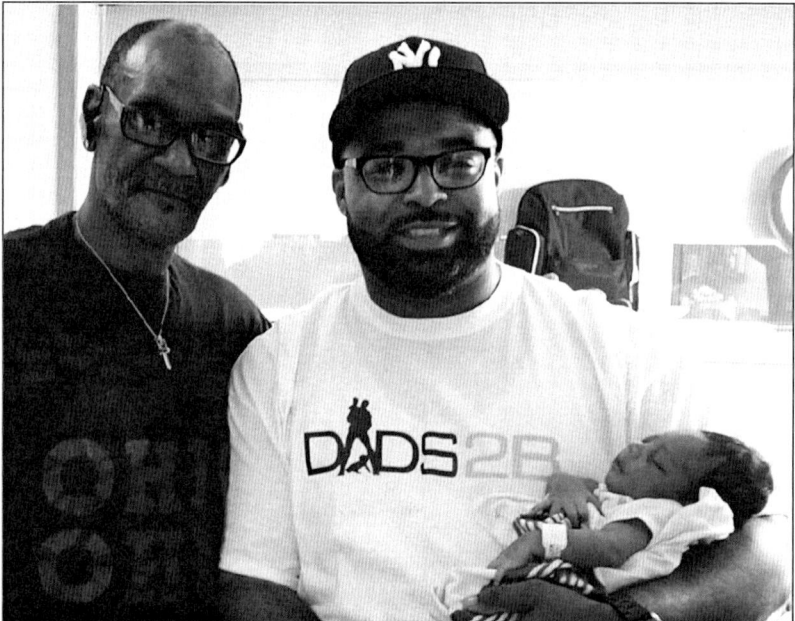

David Fluellen, right, holds a new Moms2B baby son of a Dads2B father.

Lessons Learned

- Women, infant and children all benefit from a supportive co-parenting environment that creates better mental and physical well-being and behaviors that can have lifelong benefits.
- Attracting fathers to attend a pregnancy and parenting program was successful because of the unique integration of Moms2B with Dads2B, and the positive relationships fathers developed with the staff.
- Fathers need and deserve to feel valued and involved to promote better pregnancy outcomes and to solve the Black-white disparities in infant mortality.

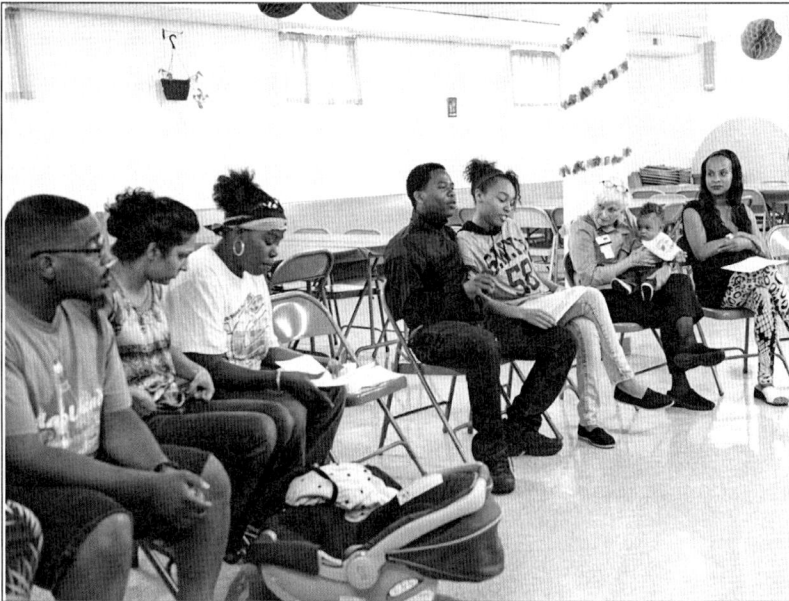

Dads join Sister-Brother Circle at Weinland Park.
(Photo by Mandy Groszko, Ohio State)

10 | Key Leaders in Fighting Infant Mortality

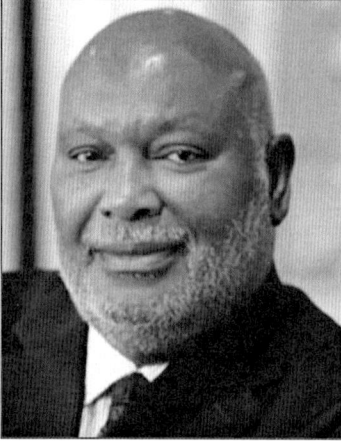

Dr. Arthur James arrived in Columbus from Kalamazoo, Michigan in 2011, a year after we opened Moms2B. The Ohio Department of Health recruited him to the state to reduce our high infant mortality rate and wide disparities in birth outcomes for Black and white babies. In Kalamazoo he had developed a clinical obstetrics and gynecology practice that included services to improve socioeconomic factors, efforts that resulted in a decrease in infant deaths.

Dr. James brought his wealth of expertise and guided our strategic plans to improve maternal and child health. He also co-directed our Ohio Collaborative to Prevent Infant Mortality. In these roles he spoke and taught throughout Ohio and at Midwest regional and national forums, explaining how centuries of legalized slavery followed by Jim Crow laws cemented racist social norms that caused and continue to fuel the disparities that remain today. He helped his audiences, and our community, better understand that differences in maternal and infant health and mortality couldn't be explained away based on factors outside of racism and persistent inequities.

He used a graph to show that the longstanding racial gaps in infant mortality rates would persist for at least 40 more years, and even then, in 2052, Black rates would only reach the federal goals achieved among white infants in 2012. Clearly, to reach equity we needed to accelerate our efforts.

Ohio Infant Mortality Rates from 1968-2020

——Black/African American

——White

——Total

········ Linear (Black/African American)

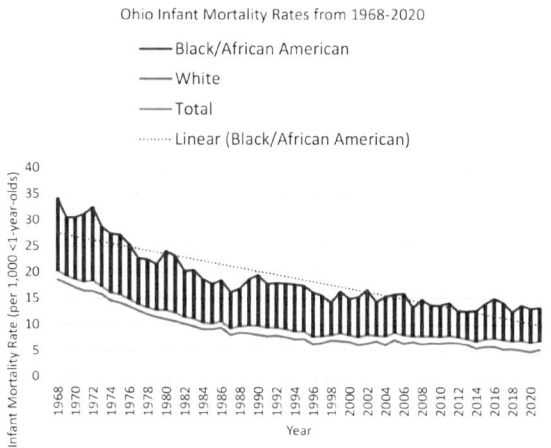

While the Black-white disparities slowly narrows over time, it remains a tragic measure of long-standing inequities. Data from Kathy Cowan, Director of Epidemiology, Columbus Public Health.

Ohio had one of the highest Black infant mortality rates in the country at the time, placing seventh nationally in number of births and ranked sixth highest for the number of infant deaths. Every year, more than 1,000 infants died in Ohio including 350 Black infants and most of their deaths occurred in nine predominantly urban counties. Armed with these facts, Dr. James convinced a group of maternal and child health professionals to select nine Ohio counties with the highest rates of disparities for the Institute for Equity in Birth Outcomes support. This gave Ohio more federal and state aid to collect data and provide resources to predominantly Black neighborhoods. Franklin County, the home of Moms2B, was one of the nine, meaning that we now had more aid to meet equity goals.[6]

To achieve equity, Dr. James explained we must "step up to keep up." This meant upstream policy changes. For those unfamiliar with upstream vs. downstream strategies, he used the parable:

a person walking downstream along a fast-moving river sees someone struggling in the water to stay alive. After he rescues one person, others come, crying for help to be rescued. Finally, the person tires of constantly rescuing people and walks upstream to discover people falling off an unprotected cliff. After conducting a successful campaign for a strong guard rail, the falls into the river stop.

At Moms2B we saw firsthand that pregnant and parenting women needed immediate help. At the time, we didn't realize that we could also help to improve their chances of health and well-being with upstream policies. Then we were introduced to two dynamic state senators.

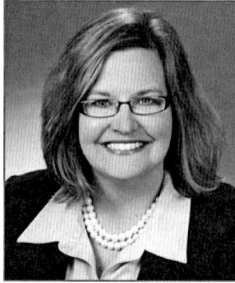

Senator Shannon Jones   Senator Charleta Tavares

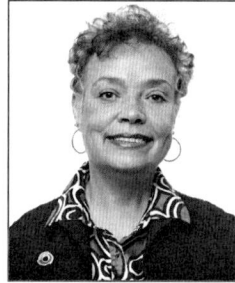

In 2013, state senators Shannon Jones and Charleta Tavares were determined to publicize Ohio's crisis in maternal and infant health and find solutions before their terms ended. They toured the state to learn more about existing programs and to hear directly from families. In Columbus, they held their public hearing at Ohio State East Hospital where they listened to stories from Moms2B participants and learned more about our model.

Afterwards, Senator Jones wrote: "It's shocking that nearly 1,000 Ohio babies die each year before their first birthday—a rate higher than many developing countries." She called the racial disparities not only "shocking," but "immoral and completely unacceptable."

"This gross inequity demands outrage from all of us... it is worthy of deep introspection, vigorous debate, and unrelenting action to change the system that is failing too many Ohio families."

Their tour resulted in 2014 legislation to create Ohio's Infant Mortality Commission. Dr. James and I were appointed to the commission and led the subgroup on the social determinants of health. We pressed for community changes, especially for safe, affordable housing.

Senator Jones called Dr. James and me to a meeting with the Ohio Housing Finance Agency. The director and staff arrived wondering why their agency was called for a meeting about infant mortality, not grasping the connection. Through stories I was able to share about Moms2B moms who struggled to find housing, putting themselves and their babies at risk, we convinced agency leaders that a stable home would improve the health of mothers and infants, provide a safe place for infants to sleep and reduce disparities. Senator Jones ended the meeting after soundly convincing the agency they needed to step up and help secure housing for pregnant women.

The senators held eight productive commission hearings and issued a report capturing key strategies for legislators to consider.

Meanwhile, more organizations joined Dr. James in his call to "step up to keep up." Soon after the Ohio Hospital Association agreed to help, their clinical director, Dr. Robert Falcone, analyzed the numbers of potential infant lives saved if specific actions were adopted.

His abbreviated list follows.

Action	Annual potential infant lives saved in Ohio
Safe sleep education, with cribs and Pack 'n Plays	74
Reduce health disparities	81
Breast milk for newborns and beyond	25
Safe Spacing of the next pregnancy	129
Access to pre, post and inter-conception care	58
Total yearly impact	367 lives saved

Initially, the association asked birthing hospitals to focus on breastmilk for newborns and teaching the ABCs of safe sleep including offering a portable crib if parents did not have a safe place for their infant to sleep. To reduce health disparities, the association urged health care providers to take diversity training that included the potential effects of racism on health care and infant mortality.

Later, the association started a Good 4 Baby statewide campaign to teach and practice safe sleep for newborns in hospital nurseries and advocate for and support breastfeeding.

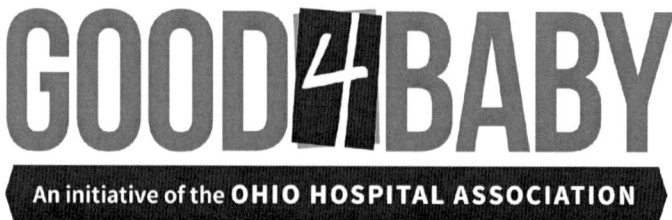

GOOD 4 BABY

An initiative of the OHIO HOSPITAL ASSOCIATION

In my view, based on obstetrics science, the most effective life-saving action on Dr. Falcone's list was safe spacing of the next pregnancy. Placement of long-acting, reversible contraceptives (LARC), such as IUDs, is the most effective way to achieve the goal of 18 to 24 months between delivery and the next pregnancy. Many professional organizations and public health agencies promoted the Ohio Collaborative efforts to make this type of birth control affordable and available to prevent teenage pregnancies and help women recover from one pregnancy before their next. One popular method was to ask, "Do you want to become pregnant in the next year?" If not, then health providers would offer suggestions, including placement of long-acting reversible contraceptives.

By 2017, legislators had shaped some of the recommendations of the Ohio Infant Mortality Commission into law. SB 332 from the 131st General Assembly (Jones and Tavares) passed with bipartisan support and the governor's blessing and, importantly, addressed housing.

Housing items included:
- The Ohio Housing Finance Agency shall include reducing infant mortality as a priority housing need in the agency's annual plan.
- The Ohio Housing Finance Agency and the Ohio Development Services Agency shall include pregnancy as a priority in its housing assistance programs and local emergency shelter programs.
- Development of a rental housing assistance program to expand housing opportunities for extremely low-income households that include pregnant women or new mothers.

Also in the law:
- Timely data with quarterly scorecards from the Department of Health and Medicaid with preterm births and infant mortality rates by race and ethnicity. Periodic reports of progress towards lowering disparities and mortality rates.
- Health care professionals must have access to education and/or experiential learning on racial inequities and their impact on health.

- Collaboration between the Department of Health and Medicaid to support reproductive health through:
  - Enrolling pregnant women into Medicaid without delay by giving them presumptive eligibility.
  - Expanding access to evidence-based home visiting. (Only 4,000 families a year were receiving home visiting services; thousands more were eligible.)
  - Smoking cessation programs.
  - Assuring long-acting reversible contraceptives (LARCs) were easily available, with mandates to hospitals to offer to place LARCs in all women who desired them after delivery and before discharge.
  - Safe sleep education for professionals and infant caretakers, assuring families have an approved crib or portable Play Yard (Pack 'n Play) for their newborns.
  - Regular scorecards that monitor reproductive and infant health including time to access Medicaid, preconception care, early entry into prenatal care, uptake of LARCs, breastfeeding, smoking, behavioral health and infant safe sleep practices — all by race, ethnicity, and region of state.

Coupled with funding and explicit legal requirements, the legislation took steps to correct centuries of inequitable social and medical treatment.

Governor Kasich and Medicaid

An important backdrop to this new law was Governor John Kasich's defiance of his party when, in 2014, he expanded Medicaid under the Affordable Care Act. Medicaid in Ohio already covered pregnant women living with incomes 200% or less of federal poverty levels. Expansion gave more than 650,000 citizens with incomes at or below 138% of poverty access to medical care. This action allowed more women to access medical care in the preconception period, ideally to treat conditions such as diabetes and hypertension before they were pregnant. With Medicaid expansion, Ohio became one of the states with the highest proportion of citizens covered by medical insurance.

SB 332 also made it easier to use the Medicaid benefit by giving women presumptive eligibility for pregnancy care to prevent the long delays they often faced in obtaining insurance coverage. This provision was championed by Medicaid Medical Director Dr. Mary Applegate, another physician aware from her own pediatric practice of how essential health insurance was for maternal and child health. With timely insurance coverage, women could receive prenatal care in their first trimester and medications such as progesterone, both of which could help prevent premature births. Other provisions in SB 332 made this process much easier.

As we learned from history and our Moms2B participants, many factors outside of medical care needed to change before we would meaningfully make a difference on the racial inequity front.

Once SB 332 reached Governor Kasich's desk, he designated $26 million more from Medicaid funds to support Equity Institute counties, a portion of which came to CelebrateOne to fund Moms2B growth and sustain our eight sites. And Medicaid offered other funds to Ohio's health care systems if they met quality measures or reached into communities with innovative projects. This money could be used to improve mental health and addiction, chronic diseases or maternal and infant health. Ohio State's health system met Medicaid's quality metrics and served a large group of patients with Medicaid insurance, enabling them to access these funds.

Our program met the criteria for an innovative community improvement project for maternal and infant health and Ohio

State leadership invited Moms2B to apply for support, which led to an essential financial lifeline.

Next came an ambitious offer from the university medical center to fulfill a dream and build a mobile clinic. After a year of careful planning, our fully equipped "Community Care Coach" opened in March 2020 with new Moms2B Medical Director Dr. Kamilah Dixon, an obstetrician-gynecologist, on board.

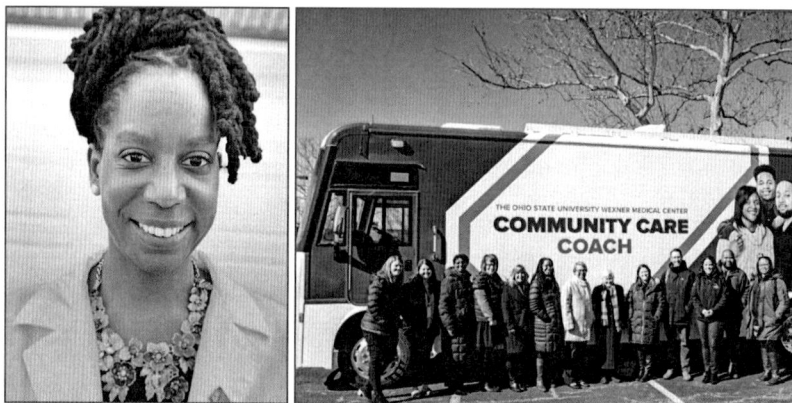

Dr. Kamilah Dixon, Moms2B Medical Director, also staffs the Community Care Coach at Moms2B North.

For the first time, pregnant and postpartum patients could receive two hours of education, emotional and material support at Moms2B and then step outside for prenatal, postpartum and reproductive health care, eliminating transportation and child-care burdens for parents and building trust in the health care system.

Colleagues from Ohio State Family Medicine shared the clinic and served other neighborhoods, making health care readily available five days a week where the need was highest.

During the COVID pandemic, the coach offered testing and vaccinations. In July 2022, as in-person Moms2B sessions partially reopened, the coach rolled out again to Moms2B North.

Governor Mike DeWine and First Lady Fran DeWine

In 2018, Fran DeWine, wife of then gubernatorial candidate Mike DeWine visited a Moms2B session in Linden. As she walked in, Twinkle handed her a baby to hold. We heard that after her visit, when she spoke across the state, she told how Moms2B reminded her of the OSU Extension group she joined as a new mother and found so helpful.

After assuming the governorship, both DeWines continued their strong support, and even asked us to bring Moms2B statewide. In March of 2020, Steve and I began that work, telling physicians and community leaders at Wright State College of Medicine about Moms2B and asking for their support and collaboration to bring Moms2B to Dayton. But as we wrapped up our community forum, we received an urgent call from Columbus. We needed to close Moms2B in-person sites. The governor had just issued emergency COVID pandemic containment orders.

Like the rest of the country and most of the world, we were forced to reimagine how we operated. Moms2B virtual began the next day as our team quickly transitioned. We also made one-on-one telephone connections and arranged drop-off sites for food, clothes and other supplies. Everyone stayed masked and socially distanced. Dr. Dixon and I published a description of our successful transition from a vibrant in-person community program to active groups in a virtual environment. A paper in Clinical Obstetrics and Gynecology, 2021 describes the steps we took.[7]

As vaccinations and treatments became available and the pandemic surge receded, Moms2B reopened in a hybrid format.

Timeline for Ohio

2011 • Dr. Arthur James recruited by Ohio State and Ohio's Department of Health to lead strategic plans and co-direct Ohio Collaborative to Prevent Infant Mortality.

2013 • State Senators Shannon Jones and Charleta Tavares tour the state to publicize and review programs that help to reduce Ohio's high infant mortality rates and disparities.

• Dr. James presses and wins Equity Institute support for nine Ohio counties to focus on eliminating disparities.

• Ohio Hospital Association joins efforts and designs Good4Baby initiatives.

2014 • Legislators create Infant Mortality Commission after Jones and Tavares tour.

• Governor John Kasich expands Medicaid under the Affordable Care Act for 650,000 Ohioans.

2015 • Infant Mortality Commission holds eight public hearings from August-December.

2016 • Ohio Commission on Infant Mortality issues report in March.

2017 • Senate Bill 332 (Jones/Tavares, 131st General Assembly) signed into law to codify multiple strategies to improve maternal and child health from the Ohio Commission report.

• Governor Kasich commits $26.8 million from Medicaid funds to improve birth outcomes and reduce disparities, benefits Moms2B.

• Ohio Department of Health increases home visiting, Help Me Grow, Community Health Workers.

2018 • Governor DeWine wins office.

2020 • In March a SARS-CoV global pandemic declared; Moms2B and Dads2B teams quickly pivot in-person sessions to successful, virtual formats in Columbus and Dayton.

11 | Come to a Moms2B Session

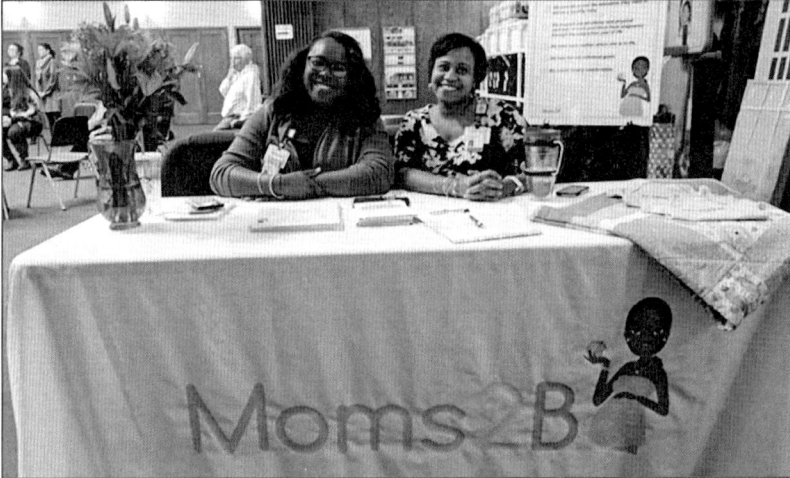

Community Health Worker LaTonya Dowdell and Social Worker Tomasina Richards welcome families and volunteers at a Moms2B open house. Attendees sign in at a table like this when they come to sessions.

I believe that at the heart of Moms2B's success is the routine and stability of a weekly touchpoint for moms and families — and the magic is in the mix of what participants experience there, not one single element. I'd like to walk you through a typical Thursday session at Moms2B East in the Wallace Auditorium of The Ohio State University East Hospital.

At this site on the Near East Side, we start at 4:30 p.m., later than other sessions, to attract families who come after typical work and school hours. This brings upwards of 50 people each week from the Near East Side, a historically predominantly Black neighborhood where premature birth and infant death rates are high. We opened this site in 2011 in response to troubling birth outcomes there.

If you come early, you will help the Moms2B team prepare, and witness how our experienced team of a dietitian, nurse educator, social worker, community health worker, health professional students, child development staff, students and volunteers organize this busy session. We'll arrange chairs for pregnant women and their partners to sit in Sister-Brother Circle in the spacious auditorium and set up chairs and spread quilts out in a smaller room for new moms and their infants. Outside the entrance, a long table will be piled high with donations — new and slightly used baby and children's clothes from generous supporters. Inside the auditorium, the hospital cafeteria staff will have arranged a table with fruits and vegetables and tanks filled with ice water for the families as they arrive.

Today's Schedule

4:30 p.m. Moms, dads, partners and children arrive, check in and have a snack.

4:45 to 5:15 p.m. Sister-Brother Circle forms, with separate groups for pregnant and parenting women.

- Pregnant women and their support people, including dads, gather in the auditorium.
- Parenting women with infants gather in another room.
- Conversation-starter Sister Circle question: **"Name one thing you can do to have a healthy pregnancy?"** or **"What is one thing you can do to relax?"**
- Colorful handouts are passed for today's short teaching topics: **Precious Proteins** and **Breathing out your Stress with Bubbles.**

5:30 to 6 p.m. Long lessons

- Pregnant Group: **Car Seat Safety: Keep our Babies Safe with a Carrier Lesson.**
- Parenting Group: **Immunizations and Well-Child Checkups.**
- **Dads: Dads2B group with a lesson from "Nurturing Father."**

6 to 6:30 p.m. Dinner together and individual check-in

6:30 p.m. Pack up to leave.

Session Flow

At the start of the session, we stand outside the entrance to Wallace Auditorium and watch a small fleet of Yellow Cabs drive up. Children jump out while a woman places her infant in a stroller then walks towards the steps where a Moms2B team member stands ready to help lift the stroller and welcome her. Another team member thanks the cab drivers and signs for the service.

More participants, along with friends and family — including a handful of dads — arrive, walking from a home nearby or in their own vehicles. Our Moms2B team welcomes them with high fives, smiles and hugs — typically greeting them by name. In many cases, moms are with us from early in their pregnancies, and our relationships can become close quickly.

As they enter the meeting room, participants sign in at a table staffed by two Moms2B team members and receive a $5 Kroger gift card and name tags. A woman who comes for the first time receives an especially warm welcome and orientation from a community health worker or another team member.

From a mom:
> *"Beyond the instant comfort I felt with the program, I was able to build long-lasting and powerful relationships. I have made lots of friends in similar situations. I have received information from nutrition specialists, doctors, nurses and workers in social agencies. They supported me through food recalls, home visits and general care. I also received $5 stipends for attending the program. These were helpful with food, gas and diapers."*

Women browse the donation table and select items for their families. Before they sit down, they fill a snack plate full of fresh fruit and vegetables and pour a cup of water for themselves and their children. If a woman arrives early, a team member does a brief checklist review:

- Do you plan to breastfeed?
- Do you have a car seat for the new baby?
- Do you plan to have another baby in the next two years?
- Do you have a safe place for baby to sleep?
  A crib or Pack 'n Play?
- Do you have primary care?
  Does your child(ren) have primary care?
- Do you have stable housing?
- Do you have WIC (Women Infant and Children's supplemental food program)?
- Do you have enough money to pay your bills this month?
- Do you have health insurance?
- Do you have enough food to get through the week?
- Do you smoke?
- Over the last two weeks how often have you felt nervous, anxious, or on edge?
- Over the last two weeks, how often have you felt unable to stop or control worrying?

Women who need help are connected to the appropriate community resources. That could mean accessing a car seat or Pack 'n Play or connecting mom or dad with a smoking cessation program. It could mean linking the mom to a counselor at Ohio State or in the community for mental health concerns. In cases where a mom needs housing or financial assistance, a social worker and/or housing advocate is brought into the conversation, either in the moment or following the meeting.

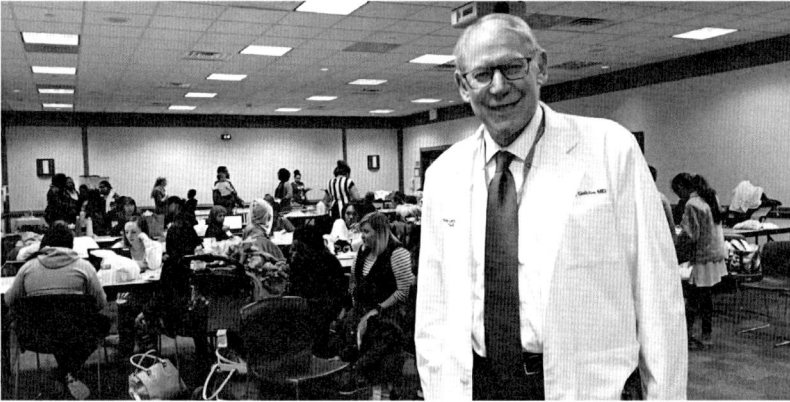
Dr. Steven Gabbe arrives weekly from the Ohio State College of Medicine to join Sister-Brother Circle. He contributes to teaching and answers questions.

One story that illustrates the importance of this partnership is one day when Steve and I arrived together and found a mom named Marie waiting for us, 24 weeks pregnant and distressed, worried that her baby was arriving already and not feeling well. Steve spoke with her, concluding that she needed to go to the hospital, and reaching out to his colleagues there to let them know she was on her way. A short time later, we heard from the obstetrician that Marie had an emergency delivery of a healthy but premature baby. Had she waited much longer — had she not come to the program that day — things could have ended much worse for mom or baby, as Marie had a fever and sepsis.

Sister-Brother Circle

After everyone gets settled, a Moms2B team leader calls together Sister-Brother Circle and directs others to their groups: "Pregnant women, stay here in the auditorium. Parenting women go with Dr. Pat. Children join Mimi and Katie in the hallway where you hear the music playing."

Because Moms2B East sessions occur in late afternoon, many school-age children also attend. One mother told me, *"I really didn't want to get the baby and myself ready to come, but my older child said I want to go to Moms2B—so we came."*

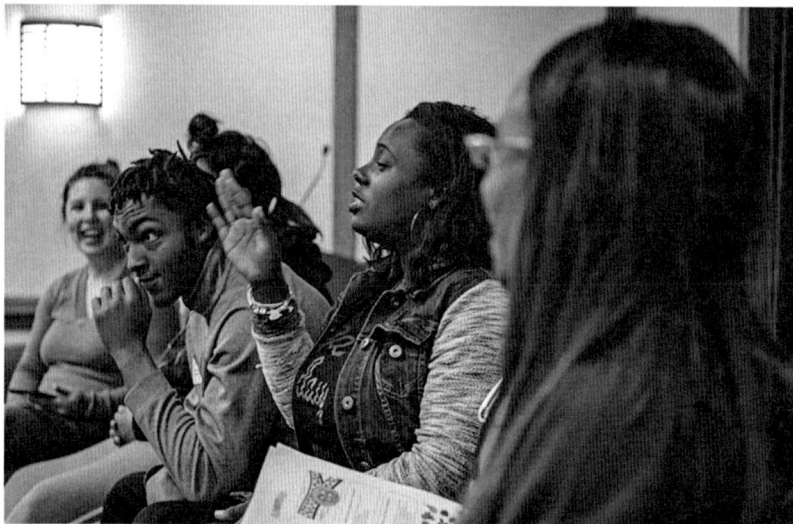

LaTonya Dowdell opens the Sister-Brother Circle pregnancy group at Moms2B East—a lesson on anemia is about to begin.

Pregnancy Group

At the start of Sister-Brother Circle, a Moms2B member introduces herself and guests. She asks each person to introduce themself, share how many weeks pregnant they are (if applicable) and answer an opening question: "Name one thing you can do this week to have a healthy pregnancy."

Some speak quietly, some with confidence. Some exude delight that they have a baby on the way, others are worried and afraid because of problems with previous pregnancies. We hear a variety of responses: Eat right, take some walks, reduce my stress, move out of the neighborhood, find a new home, stop fighting with my man, stop smoking, go to my clinic appointments. It's in these moments where trust is built, where confidences are shared. It's a sacred part of our program and, I believe, central to our team's ability to meaningfully work with our moms and dads to explore their vulnerabilities, celebrate their joy and create the kind of small community that can make a tremendous difference at the beginning of a new life.

When the circle arrives at the new mom, the team leader says, "Let's welcome Iris and clap her into our group" and hearty applause follows.

Next, our dietitian circulates a handout on the topic for the week. Today, she talks about precious proteins, first asking everyone to call out their favorite protein. After this lesson, our social worker passes out bubble water with a wand to teach an exercise called breathing out your stress. Last week she spoke about anxiety and used the handout seen here. Today, she offers a way to relax to reduce stress that may lead to anxiety attacks.

She says, "As a parent, it can be hard to find time to relax. Find ways to turn everyday activities into a way to unwind. The key is being purposeful," and shares the following handout.

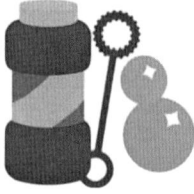

1. Begin by taking a couple of deep breaths in through your nose, exhaling slowly through your mouth
2. Think about a worry that is bothering you.
3. Breath in slowly, as deeply as you can.
4. As you exhale, visualize blowing the worry into the bubble.
5. Picture the worry inside the bubble.
6. Watch as it floats away and pops, carrying the worry far, far from you.
7. Know that the worry has popped and is outside of you now, unable to bother you anymore.
8. Keep blowing bubbles until you feel calmer and more relaxed.

"Use this activity as a fun way to teach your child how to do calm breathing. They will relax as you practice the activity. Talk to them about using the technique on their own when they are feeling anxious or upset," she says.

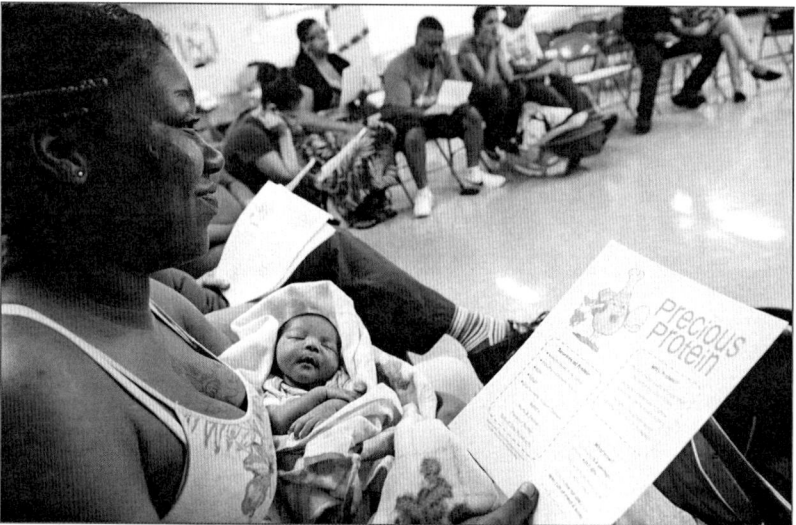

A mom with a newborn participates in parenting circle at Weinland Park.

Parenting Group

Today the parenting circle is led by a community health worker who introduces herself, telling the group she has a Moms2B child, and welcomes a new mom who is cuddling her newborn. The mom arrives to claps and congratulations. The question of the day for the parents is: "What is one thing you do to relax?" We hear: take a walk, listen to music, take a shower or a bath, do housework, practice mindfulness. The dietitian and social worker join the parenting group to teach about protein and stress reduction. The children especially love the bubble breathing exercise and take the bubble makers home at the end of session.

Nearby, child development specialists and student volunteers care for infants on quilts spread on the floor near their parents. Infants receive developmentally appropriate gross motor exercises, sensory stimulation and fine motor play with toys.

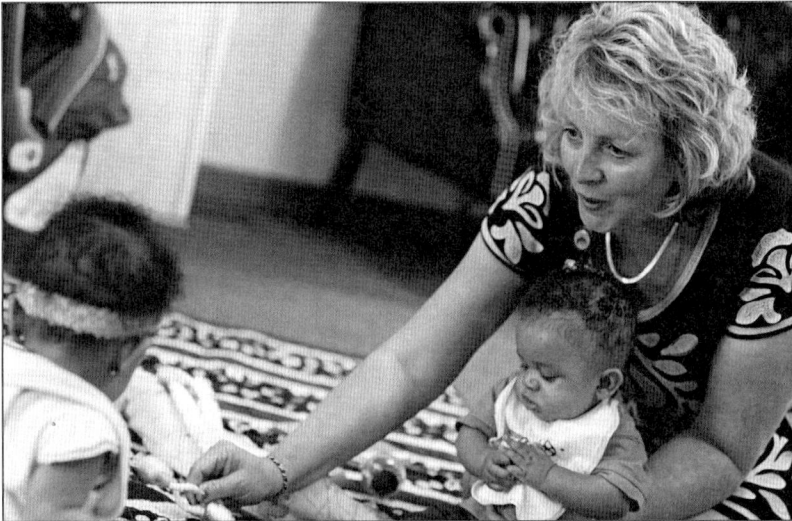

Twinkle Schottke, co-director and later director of Moms2B, kneeling, models age-appropriate activities for infants while parents participate in lessons nearby. This photo comes from Moms2B South.

Large Lesson for the Parenting Group

In the parenting room, our nurse educator teaches infant well checks and immunizations to prepare families for the Nationwide Children's Mobile Clinic next week. She encourages parents to bring their children onto the unit staffed by a pediatrician or nurse practitioner to check an illness or update immunizations and well checks.

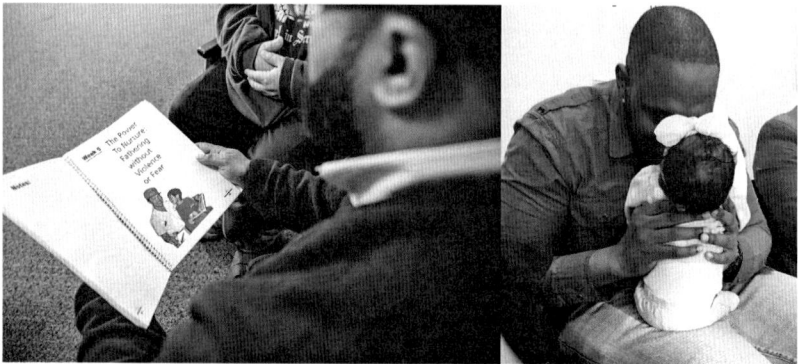

A father holds his baby girl as David Fluellen prepares to lead a group of Dads2B.

Dads2B

After dads finish the Sister-Brother Circle lessons they join David Fluellen for a group discussion. After the session, Dads2B Navigator Louis Pollard helps connect dads to jobs and resources they need to support their families.

Large Lesson for the Pregnancy Group

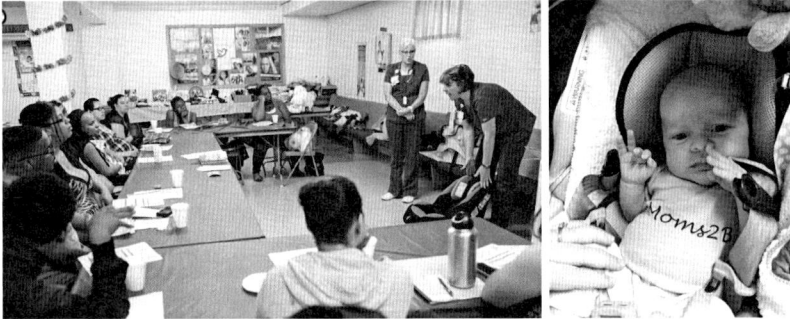

The large lesson today will be car seat safety. Dawn and Jo, Mount Carmel Welcome home nurses explain that pregnant women need their infant seats ready to go when they deliver because hospitals require it before discharge. Installation and proper fit require careful training, which most members of the Moms2B team have.

Dinner and Wrap Up

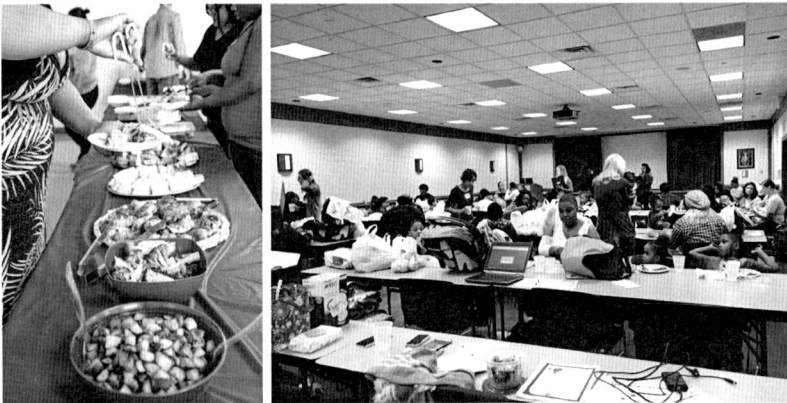

After the lessons wrap up, dinner arrives from the cafeteria. Everyone helps themselves — pregnant women first — and settles at the long tables to eat and talk. Staff work the crowd, laptops in hand, to do a final individual check-in reviewing immediate needs and long-term goals. Volunteers distribute donations, including diapers and wipes.

Planning for the Week Ahead

After the session ends, the Moms2B team packs up, reorganizes the room and makes notes on the families who need discussion at a team meeting and follow-up during the week ahead.

Lessons Learned

- Practicing Twinkle's CPR — being consistent, predictable, and reliable — is the foundation of Moms2B.
- Team members are the key to success.
- Families come and return because they know they will be warmly welcomed, respected and their voices will be heard.
- Families know they will receive teaching materials that are interactive and trustworthy from an experienced professional team during the sessions; they will receive material goods that meet their needs and follow-up after sessions.

12 | Moms2B Matters: Measuring our Impact

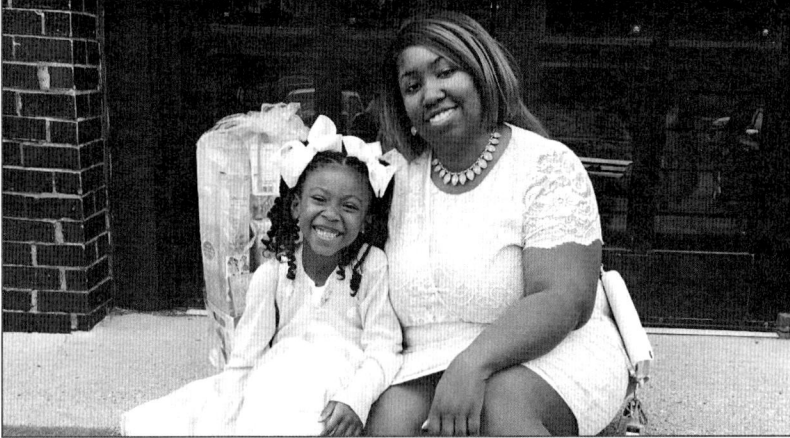

"Hello Dr. Pat, I have been thinking about you and I just wanted to say that I am grateful and will be forever grateful for Moms2B. It has been 7 years now since you all have made an impact on my life. All is well. My daughter that you and Moms2B helped nurture is attending school. I am working for the last five years and finishing my associate and bachelor's degree from Franklin University. You all were my support, my everything at a time when I needed it and I will always hold that close to my heart. Peace and Blessings to you all."

–Kateresa Lee

Feeling the power of deep connections in Sister Circle, hearing from individual moms about the lasting impact of their experiences, seeing the good that can come from one-on-one check-ins with social workers, doctors and nutritionists — I don't discount any of that. But as a researcher and scientist, as someone mindful of how we are spending scarce community dollars in our efforts, I am keenly aware that the data matters, and matters a lot.

At this stage in the story of Moms2B, it's important to attempt to answer some key questions. Did we meet our goals to improve birth outcomes with fewer low birthweight infants, fewer preterm births and fewer infant deaths? Did we contribute to the education and development of new health care providers who better understand how social determinants contribute to birth outcomes and infant mortality?

By 2014, we had taught, recruited, nurtured, designed, revised and finally created a solid Moms2B program. We had expanded to three more neighborhoods, reached 421 women, and spent almost a million dollars. To measure our impact, we looked at our first neighborhood, Weinland Park, an area comprising thirty square blocks and two census tracts and where we started in 2010. Data collected at Moms2B from 2011 through 2014 combined with analysis of vital statistics records from Columbus Public Health and data from the Ohio Medicaid program gave us a striking and encouraging picture.

In an article published in 2017 in the Maternal and Child Health Journal, we described our innovative interdisciplinary program that promoted healthy nutrition, provided social and medical support, encouraged women to breastfeed, and promoted safe sleep and healthy spacing of pregnancies.[8] We found that moms in the program appeared to act on our teaching and support. More breastfed (76%) their infants than their peers who did not attend Moms2B. Those with repeat pregnancies often waited at least 18 months until their next pregnancy. Most importantly, there were no infant deaths during this time among babies born to moms who attended the Weinland Park Moms2B program.

By comparison, six infants in the neighborhood died in the four years before Moms2B opened in Weinland Park and one infant whose mother did not attend the program died in the four years after we established a presence in the neighborhood. We concluded that our program contributed to a nearly five-fold reduction in infant mortality in Weinland Park — from 14.2 to 2.9 per 1,000 live births.

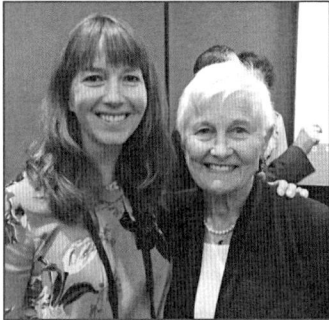

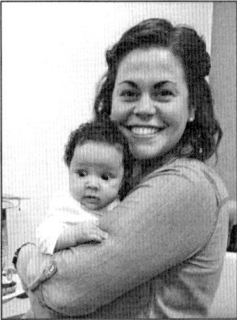

Rebecca (Becky) Reno on the left with me and Carmen Clutter on the right. Becky and Carmen were Ohio State students who co-authored our first paper.

Improving Maternal and Infant Child Health Outcomes with Community-Based Pregnancy Support Groups: Outcomes from Moms2B Ohio

Patricia Temple Gabbe[1] · Rebecca Reno[1] · Carmen Clutter[1] · T. F. Schottke[1] · Tanikka Price[1] · Katherine Calhoun[1] · Jamie Sager[1] · Courtney D. Lynch[2]

In Weinland Park the infant death rate declined almost five-fold after Moms2B was established.

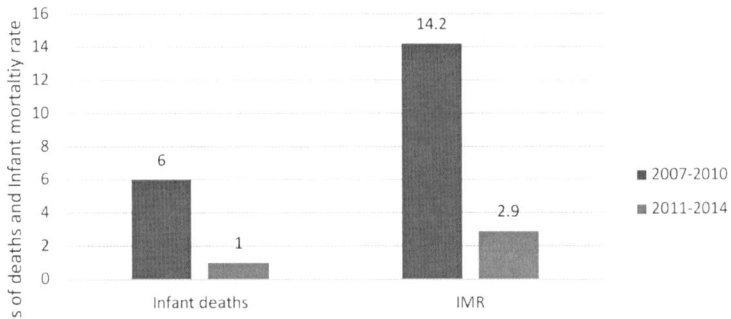

IMR=Infant Mortality Rate, the Number of Infant Deaths/1000 births
There were no deaths to women attending Moms2B

Fortunately, deaths declined even though the percentage of babies born early and at low birthweights persisted, alongside a surprisingly high percentage (13%) of twin births and one set of triplets. Twin and triplet infants often deliver early, and Black triplets experience extremely high infant death rates. The great news: the twins and triplets within our program thrived.

In another group of 56 women attending Moms2B, then Ohio State student Becky Reno found more evidence that our teachings increased moms' understanding of the benefits of breastfeeding. In her study, 80% breastfed in the hospital. Almost half of the women said they had difficulties and needed more support but did not request it. To fill this need, more of our staff became certified lactation counselors and helped women through the rough first weeks, allowing them to meet their personal goals to breastfeed for at least six months.

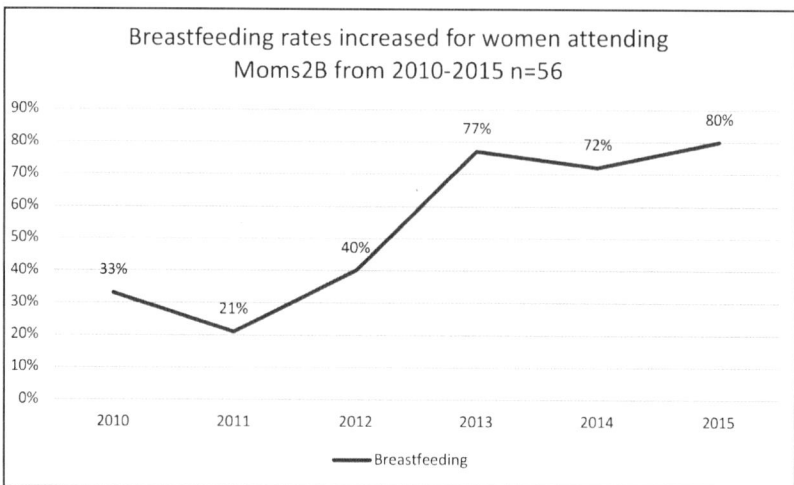

Breastfeeding rates increased for women attending
Moms2B from 2010-2015 n=56

Year	Breastfeeding
2010	33%
2011	21%
2012	40%
2013	77%
2014	72%
2015	80%

Becky Reno, then a PhD student, interviewed women attending Moms2B and found breastfeeding during the delivery hospitalization increased from 33% in 2010 to 80% in 2015. (Data and graph from Becky Reno, recreated by me).

Even five and six years after they graduated from Moms2B, mothers recalled the lessons they learned about breastfeeding. One told then MPH student Misti Crane:

> "There was a lady ...she talked about breastfeeding, she wouldn't really drill it into you, she more just gave facts and was more down to earth about it. I didn't breastfeed my daughter, but I retained a lot of information that she gave, and I ended up breastfeeding with my future babies because of that...it was more like hey, did you know, like random things about the immune system that you could pass on immunity through your breast milk."

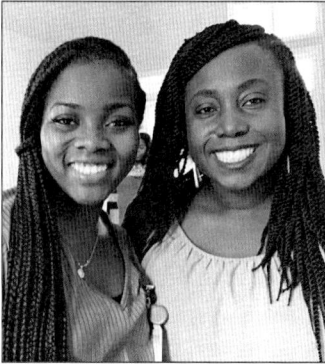

A text message from a mom:
"I just wanted to thank you again. I had spoke with probably 4 lactation nurses and still couldn't get my baby to latch until YOU helped me. I was able to stop using the shields almost immediately and she has latched ever since that exact day. My anxiety and depression about her eating has gone completely away. I can't brag enough how the entire Moms2B team has helped me in so many ways I can't count."

In a recent message seen above, a new mother struggling to breastfeed thanked Moms2B nurse Leisa Boakye-Dankwah, pictured on the right with Moms2B social work intern Crystal Vincent.

Other lessons we taught, especially around safe sleep, undoubtedly saved lives, though the impact is hard to measure.

A mother interviewed by Misti Crane said:

> "I was putting my daughter on her stomach. Even though the hospital said (to put her on her back), they don't really tell you too much about it. Like they more so explained to me there, at Moms2B, and then I stopped doing that and I haven't done it with my other ones. I knew they said it was bad in the hospital, but I didn't really know why or what or anything."

At the time of our first study, Ohio State student Tejas Venkat-Ramani wrote her honors thesis about Moms2B. Investigating causes of infant deaths, she noted the high toll of sleep related deaths in Franklin County. In two years, 67 infants died of sleep related causes. Many were found sleeping in an adult bed, a couch or chair — all known to pose suffocation risks — even though a crib or bassinet was in the home.

Over the years, through our work, the work of other advocates in the community and a concerted effort to increase public awareness around safe sleep, sleep related deaths declined in our county.

To rigorously examine the effects of our program beyond the impact in Weinland Park, our research colleagues conducted a study of 675 women who attended at least two sessions (most attended six) and gave birth from 2011 to 2017. These women then were paired with two other women who had similar characteristics but did not attend Moms2B.

Overall, when the 2,011 women in the study were compared to other pregnant individuals in Franklin County, the group faced medical and societal conditions that put them at higher risk for a premature or low birthweight infant or an infant death. Fewer had completed high school, more had a history of poor birth outcomes with more premature births. Before they became pregnant, twice as many women had high blood pressure and/or diabetes; more (34%) smoked and more were obese (35%). Most women in the study were Black (72%) and most (79%) lived in neighborhoods designated at risk because of crime, unemployment, lower educational attainment and high infant mortality rates.

This study appeared in the Maternal and Child Health Journal in 2021.[9]

Attendance at Moms2B Reduces Infant Deaths by 55%

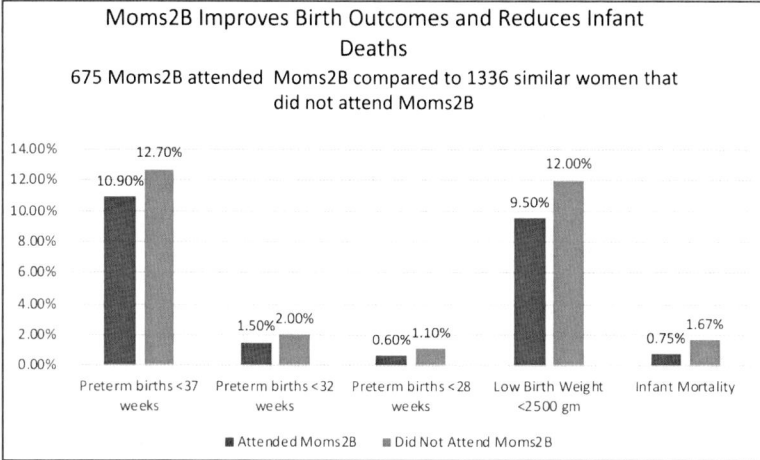

Moms2B Improves Birth Outcomes and Reduces Infant Deaths

675 Moms2B attended Moms2B compared to 1336 similar women that did not attend Moms2B

	Preterm births <37 weeks	Preterm births <32 weeks	Preterm births <28 weeks	Low Birth Weight <2500 gm	Infant Mortality
Attended Moms2B	10.90%	1.50%	0.60%	9.50%	0.75%
Did Not Attend Moms2B	12.70%	2.00%	1.10%	12.00%	1.67%

The research confirmed Moms2B as an evidence-based program to reduce the risk of preterm and low birthweight infants, especially those born extremely preterm, from 20-28 weeks. Five infants born to women attending Moms2B died, compared to 22 infants in the comparison group. In both groups, deaths occurred because of extreme prematurity, congenital anomalies or were sleep related.

A mother reported to Misti Crane:

"I would think that (safe sleep instruction) was a key point that I took away (from Moms2B) because I breastfed, so it was easy for me to just fall asleep with my child...It just made me more aware and go ahead and put them where they need to be instead of going ahead and co-sleeping."

Besides our teaching, modeling and encouragement, Mount Carmel Welcome Home nurses also reinforced how to keep infants safe from sleep related deaths when they did home visits. Even then, one infant in our study born to a woman attending Moms2B died of sleep related causes.

While we could measure birth outcomes and cost savings, there were intangibles we could not quantify. Dr. Johanna DeStefano a retired Ohio State professor, wanted to help with the infant mortality crisis in Columbus and, after we told her about Moms2B, she gave us a generous donation. Besides her monetary gift, she volunteered to join

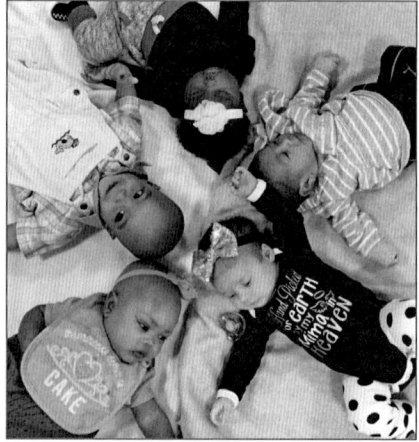

Babies at Moms2B Franklinton.

our Advisory Board, where she urged us to do more qualitative studies and collect the stories from the women who came to Moms2B.

Misti Crane, a former journalist and editor of this book who was earning her Master of Public Health answered with her culminating project, pilot research titled "Moms2B: Beyond the First Birthday." She randomly selected nine women who attended Moms2B from 2013 to 2014 to interview in the pursuit of understanding what, if any, lasting mark the program left on their lives and those of their children. Each transcribed interview reveals the trauma women had endured and brought with them to Moms2B. They tell of their deep love for their children, who were five and six years old at the time of the interviews, and how Moms2B influenced how they parent and, in some cases, helped to shape their futures. In the interviews, they recalled the warmth, respect and welcoming atmosphere from the Moms2B team and how often they helped with material and emotional support. While most women continued to thrive and meet their goals, a few had self-doubts and still coped with trauma-related mental health issues.

"There was never enough food at the shelter, I had a lot of swelling and dehydration. I was in and out of the hospital because I was always not eating and giving my portions to my kids." (She was pregnant and had three older children.) "So, they (Moms2B) gave me bags of non-perishable items to keep in my room so that I was eating something."

One woman came to Moms2B while she was in Choices, a shelter for abused women. She related how both organizations helped her recognize the signs of unhealthy relationships, ones that could lead to abuse.

Another mother said:

"They were so helpful to me. I got postpartum depression and they (Moms2B) were right there for that. I was able to tell them. I got to a point where I didn't have shoes without holes in the bottom. They ended up providing three different pairs of shoes, a dressy pair and sandals and tennis shoes. Whatever I needed, they were right there. They had so much information it was just nice. I wasn't getting home-cooked meals all the time, because with a newborn it's hard. Sitting down to a meal there, and just talking, just the support that I received there was amazing."

One mother enrolled at Columbus State and received an accounting degree. She made a good income and had employer-based health insurance. This, she said, kept her off the state's Medicaid program.

"I probably would have never gotten to where I am today if it wasn't for the foundation that they gave me and told me that I could do anything regardless of what I was dealing with, whatever I wanted to do I could do.

Another mother said:

> *"My confidence level is a lot higher than it was. Me being able to also trust people was another important part of that as well – trust that they actually would help…Being at Moms2B and really finding that they were able to help us the best way that they could, it really allowed me to have a sense of peace."*

> *"I think it's impacted my life in a way where I'm able to be a better mom for my kids because first of all being in a group that showed support and love to moms whether single or married, you know, and I think just having that support system there was the overall thing that gave me confidence to continue being a really good mother for my kids and for my household."*

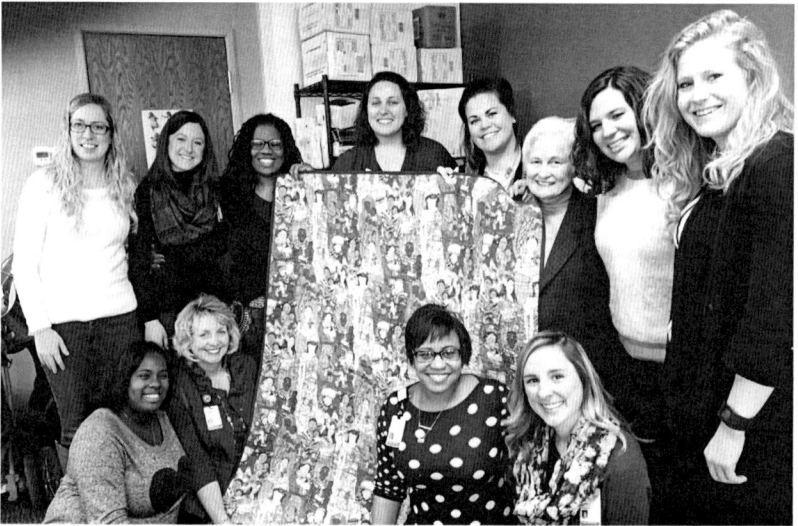

Our team displays a quilt made for Moms2B by Linda Overman, from Kazel Carbone's Church.

These interviews were reassuring, helping us to see how our team's compassion, understanding, respect and kindness made a lasting difference, and confirming our sense that the trust we built with moms in our program was vital to its success.

One woman was unable to get to a session, was home depressed and crying, and Moms2B staff went to her home and spoke with her to help her over this rough spot. Other moms recalled the help they received with items they needed but could not afford: car seats, Pack 'n Plays, diapers, wipes, healthy meals and food to take home.

The women also spoke of long-lasting benefits of techniques they learned to help them navigate parenthood and relationship challenges.

Other thoughts that women shared years after participating in Moms2B included:

"I remember (a Moms2B team member) did this whole thing where she said, 'You can't pour from an empty cup,' where she gives you the visual demonstration. So, I've kind of put that into my kids too, my 4-year-old, I'm like, hey, you've gotta kind of take a minute. Kids need a minute too."

"It's also contributed to the fact that me and my kids volunteer twice a month. We go to different soup kitchens on different holidays. Each of my kids keep a toy underneath the tree and leave it wrapped and we take it down to one of the shelters at Christmas. It really has taught me to give back."

"It taught me not to be judgmental, I guess. So, I don't let my kids live in a judgmental world and I try my best not to judge others."

One of my own memories comes from a Thursday at Moms2B at Ohio State East Hospital when a woman breastfeeding her two-week-old infant approached me and said: *"Dr. Pat I need your help. I just got an eviction notice to be out in two weeks. I have my 4-year-old son and my new baby."* She shared that her landlord worked with her, but that she was now several months behind because she couldn't work due to her high-risk pregnancy.

She told me she had worked 11 months at a long-term care facility — one month shy of receiving maternity benefits and, with the money she had saved, she paid her car and insurance payments but had nothing left for rent. In the next few days, I reached Michael Wilkos at the Columbus Foundation. He found funds through a Helping Hand grant and contacted the landlord directly to arrange for her to keep her apartment. Recently, at a community meeting, she came to me with a big smile, wearing a CelebrateOne T-shirt.

> *"Remember me Dr. Pat? You helped me with my rent, then you told me to fill out the Community Health Worker Training application and I did it on the Moms2B computer just an hour before the deadline. And they accepted me!"*

Now she worked for CelebrateOne, the Columbus organization that leads citywide efforts to address the social determinants of health, including housing, that can contribute to infant mortality.

We also saw some confirmation of our program's longer-term impact in Columbus Public Schools' kindergarten readiness level report in 2017. Seven years after Moms2B opened, children from Weinland Park were near the top of the charts for kindergarten readiness.

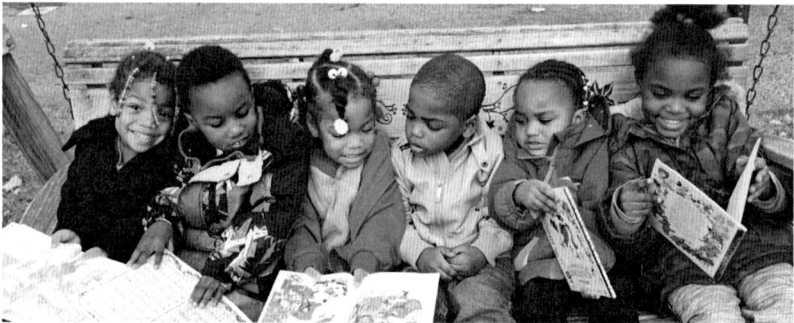

Moms2B graduates in Weinland Park reading and enjoying their books. Three of these children are the healthy triplets described in this chapter.

Kindergarten Readiness in Weinland Park
Tops Most Columbus Schools (2017)

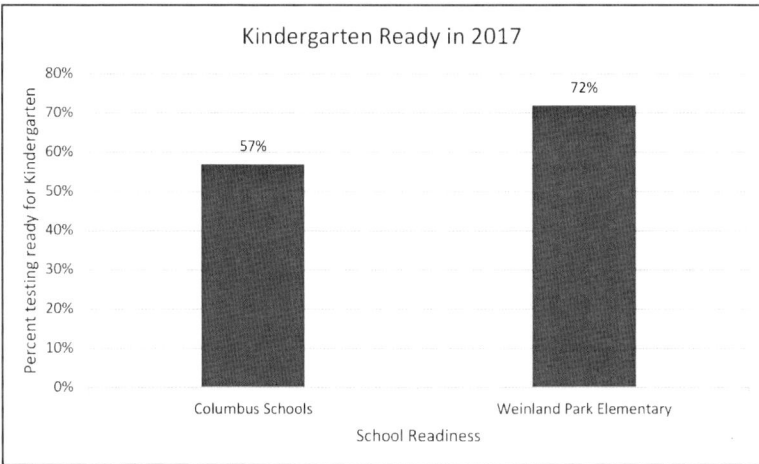

Kindergarten Ready in 2017

Columbus Schools: 57%
Weinland Park Elementary: 72%

Percent testing ready for Kindergarten (Y-axis: 0% to 80%)

School Readiness (X-axis)

Breastfeeding may enhance intelligence and cognition, another possible explanation of why Weinland Park babies start reading early and enter kindergarten better prepared.

At What Cost?

Operating expenses mounted as the number of sites opened and attendance grew.

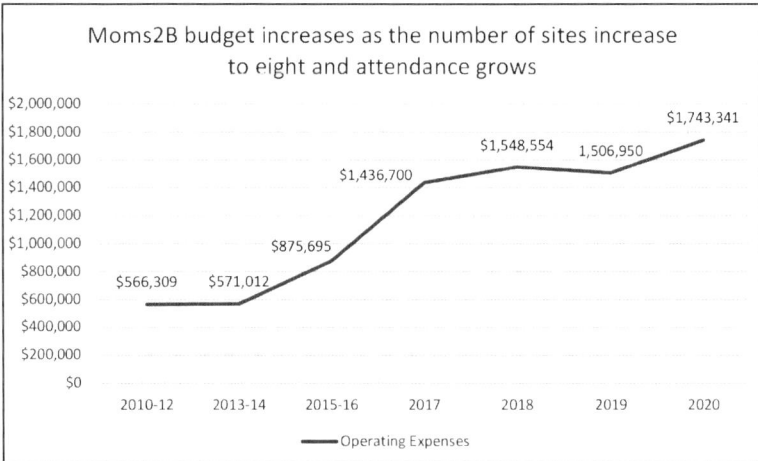

Moms2B budget increases as the number of sites increase to eight and attendance grows

2010-12: $566,309
2013-14: $571,012
2015-16: $875,695
2017: $1,436,700
2018: $1,548,554
2019: 1,506,950
2020: $1,743,341

— Operating Expenses

Cost is another data point I've kept my eye on throughout Moms2B. By 2018, we operated eight Moms2B sites at $180,000 per site. The budget paid the salaries and benefits of our team members, the cost of renting our office and the space used for our sessions, and items for the moms including transportation costs, gift cards, diapers, car seats, Pack 'n Plays, breastfeeding items and meals.

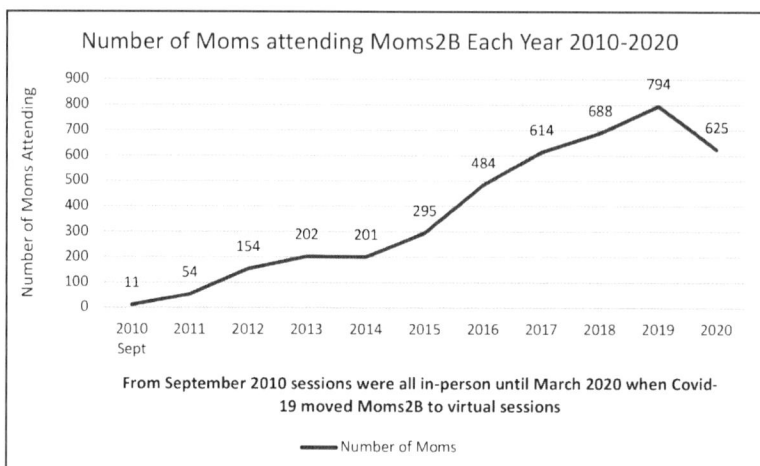

Number of Moms attending Moms2B Each Year 2010-2020

From September 2010 sessions were all in-person until March 2020 when Covid-19 moved Moms2B to virtual sessions

Over the first 10 years we spent more than $8.2 million dollars —largely through dollars provided by community partners highlighted earlier in this book. We've been mindful throughout this effort of the financial return on investment in addition to the health and other benefits we're able to measure.

Each year we invested $2,000 per woman who attended Moms2B. If we take the average hospital costs for delivery, grouped by gestational age, and compare the costs for the 675 women attending Moms2B with women who did not attend, we can calculate a rough estimate of losses or savings. Using average hospital maternal and newborn costs, published by Cincinnati Children's Hospital researchers Eric Hall and James Greenberg,[10]

I calculated average costs per infant in these gestational groups:

Gestational age at birth	Average Hospital Costs
Full-term infant 37-41 weeks	$ 3,600
Gestational age 32-36 weeks	$ 14,638
Gestational age 28-32 weeks	$127,837
Gestational age 23-28 weeks	$412,190

In comparison to women not attending Moms2B, an average of $754 was saved for each woman who attended, largely a result of fewer costly preterm births. Benefits and savings accrue for each gestational week prolonged. Adults who were born premature also face the odds of lower annual incomes ranging from $9,300 earned per year for those born extremely premature, to more than $100,000 earned per year for infants born close to term.

But How Do You Put a Price on This?

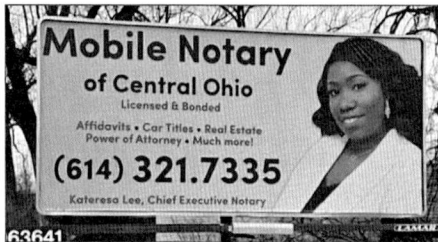

Riding along Fifth Avenue in 2020, I saw this billboard with Moms2B graduate Kateresa Lee, who is now a college-educated entrepreneur advertising her mobile notary service.

Lessons Learned
- Objective measures of Moms2B were critical and demonstrated quantitative and qualitative benefits.
- Independent analysis found that attendance at Moms2B improves infant birth outcomes and reduces the risk of an infant dying in neighborhoods in Columbus.
- Interviews of moms years after they attended Moms2B sessions found they incorporated the teachings that enhanced their lives and those of their children.
- Our program proved cost effective.

13 | Race, Racism and Our Team

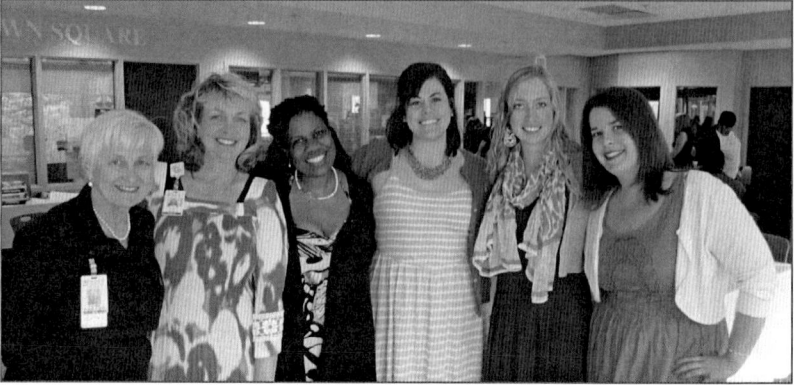

Our First Moms2B Team: Me, Twinkle Schottke, Tanikka Price, Carmen Clutter, Jamie Sager, Katie Calhoun.

Early in our program development, I was told that some people questioned why two white women thought they could create a program primarily designed to support Black women. I can understand that reflex to question, to wonder if this project was one of those where well-intentioned outsiders swoop in, confident they understand the needs of the community and try to implement a predetermined program. There are countless examples in the U.S. and abroad of work described as *for* a community closing out that community's voices, or not listening closely enough to them.

At one public panel held at Ohio State's Kirwan Institute, someone pointedly asked me: "Why don't you let Black women solve the infant mortality crisis?" I shared that it was my hope that as the community became more aware of the disparities, and of the high rates of preventable Back infant deaths, that more of the community's Black leaders and scholars would team with us in our efforts.

We remained aware that our team was primarily made up of white women, and were heartened in the early months that Moms2B appeared to be attracting moms and that many of those moms had developed strong relationships with us. Respect, listening and trust were core to our values and I believe that was key to overcoming community apprehension.

But we also wanted Black families who attended to see and learn from a team that reflected their culture and experiences and worked to diversify the Moms2B team — seeking out Black students, interns, professionals and volunteers.

Early in our program we heard Tanikka Price tell her story at a Moms2B session in Weinland Park. She had grown up in a Black family in Columbus, attended college and had given birth and nursed her first child while a college student. She earned a law degree while she raised a successful family, and she loved to teach and promote the value of education. We were able to recruit Tanikka to our team on an ongoing basis, and her contributions — in part because she was from the primary community we aimed to serve — were invaluable both to participants and to the rest of her colleagues. I was grateful that when I said something that missed the mark, something that was clearly from my white experience, she'd correct me with a smile and firm guidance: "Dr. Pat, no, no, no, you got it wrong," and then point to the back of her hand for Black or palm of her hand for white, a shorthand system we had for keeping our conversations on the right path even when we were in a larger group.

She taught, usually in Sister Circle, from her life experiences, when she had small children and little money. For example, she gave a lesson at Christmas about meaningful memories that come from experiences, not material things, like taking the children to see Christmas lights, going to the library, reading stories, singing and listening to music together. She also shared how to get gifts from Toys for Tots and other programs, including ours. When we taught reproductive health, she told what her grandmother taught her: "Don't go to bed with a man unless he's the one you want to be the father of your baby."

When one of the moms lashed out at our team for some matter, Tanikka interrupted and said: "Remember, this team does not have to be here, they are taking time from their families to help you."

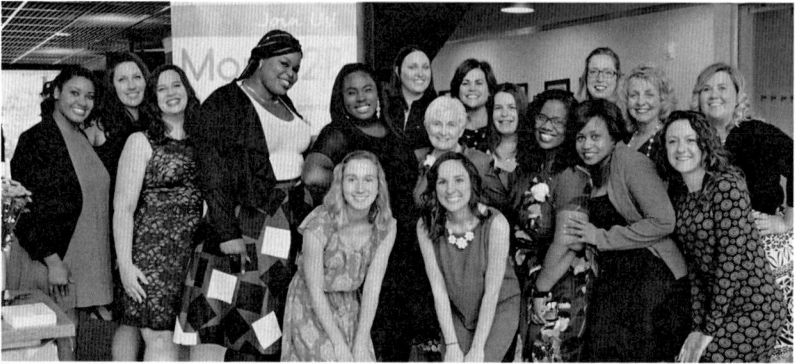

Our Moms2B team not only taught and mentored our Moms2B families, but they also planned and staffed our evening annual fundraiser, shown here at the Ohio State's Nationwide & Ohio Farm Bureau 4-H Center in 2017.

As we expanded, more Black professional women joined our team and we encouraged Moms2B graduates to train as community health workers and become part of our team. They helped us with outreach and by telling their own Moms2B stories, stepped in to lead Sister-Brother Circles and attended community events.

Recently I met a Moms2B graduate who lived in the Ohio State Scholars House for single parents and attended Ohio State. Nahla Walker asked specifically about Teeya, a Black Moms2B graduate and trained community health worker who led Sister-Brother Circle at Moms2B East where they both attended every week. She shared that Teeya, as a peer, helped her most of all.

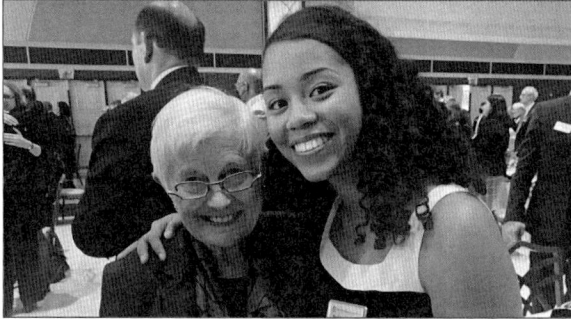

Me with Nahla Walker, a Moms2B graduate, at a Ohio State University dinner 2021.

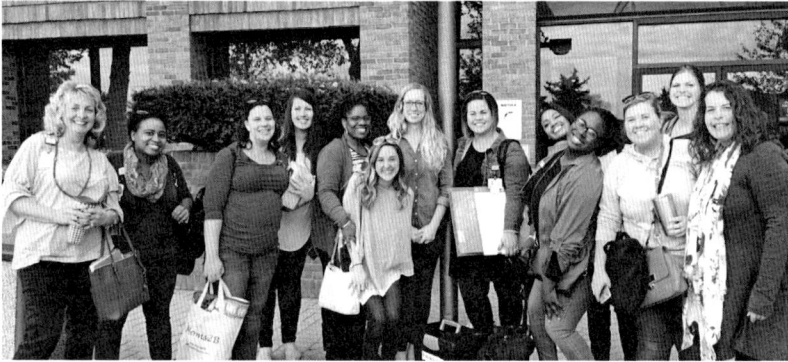

Our team prepares to enter our new office at Chatham Lane in Columbus, with a welcoming landlord and room for storage. We stayed through 2022.

In the past several years, with the nation more focused on racism, violent extremism and the systemic barriers to success that people of color experience routinely, I found myself thinking more deeply about Moms2B's connections to, and work to combat, racism as a public health crisis. I couldn't have articulated it this way when I first began to talk to colleagues about the idea of Moms2B all those years ago, but at its core it was created to fight inequity, tear down barriers and provide meaningful support. I believe it has succeeded, and hope that its impact will grow in the years to come.

On June 9, 2020, at the urging of Ohio Sen. Hearcel Craig, I submitted a written proponent testimony for Senate Concurrent Resolution 14 to declare racism a public health crisis in Ohio. I titled my testimony "I See Racism Every Day." In part, I wrote:

> *How do I "see racism?" I see it in the disparities in infant deaths in our neighborhoods, in our cities, and in our state. From our Moms and Dads in Moms2B, we learn the hard reality of why disparities exist. We see repeated evictions that uproot families and prevent children from sleeping and learning in a safe environment. We hear about the impact of hunger and lack of access to good, healthy food while pregnant. We hear how losing a job while pregnant, without maternity benefits, leads directly to an eviction and the homeless shelter. How taking two hours on public transportation can make you late for a job, or for an appointment and cause you to lose your job. Yes, this does happen in white families too. But, for Black families there has been structural discrimination for generations. There have been real estate covenants, banks redlining and freeways built through once vibrant neighborhoods. All of these stressful, local events directly affect the health of our Black families.*

> *Why disparities in infant deaths? Today, Black babies bear the burden of generations of stress and unequal treatment. They are too often born early, they struggle to breathe in our hospital NICU's, they start life at a disadvantage. They live in poorer neighborhoods, move more often into a homeless shelter, go to poorer schools, hobbled with disabilities from prematurity. They grow up with the same chronic conditions as their parents, through no fault of their own.*

> *Structural racism can be torn down; implicit racism takes time; I remember my own implicit bias. Even though I am determined to eliminate disparities, I did not know the extent of the anger, the unfair treatment, and attitudes of those that feel superior; I did not realize the fear Black families feel when they send their Black sons*

and daughters out into their neighborhoods. I believed, as most of my friends and colleagues that discrimination was in the past. I believed that by electing a Black president and First Lady we could say "there is no racism" in America; but we all saw George Floyd's murder and Ahmaud Arbery chased down for a "citizens' arrest."

I have seen how our own Moms2B and Dads2B programs have eliminated disparities in infant deaths. We have lowered infant death rates. I see, to paraphrase the great orator, Fredrick Douglass, we can grow healthy children and we must grow healthy children; this is the only way to heal the broken man and to heal our public health crisis.

This testimony reflects my own growth — my discovery years after I began work to help improve birth outcomes for Black moms and babies that we were really fighting against ongoing threats brought on by the persistent tentacles of racial hatred, tentacles that stretch back to this country's history enslaving Black people, of tearing Black families apart, of fighting a civil war to keep them in chains and working since to undermine their success and well-being.

To have co-led an organization that worked against these forces has been my great privilege.

14 | Reflections and Hopes

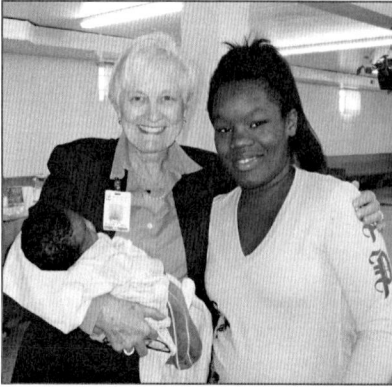

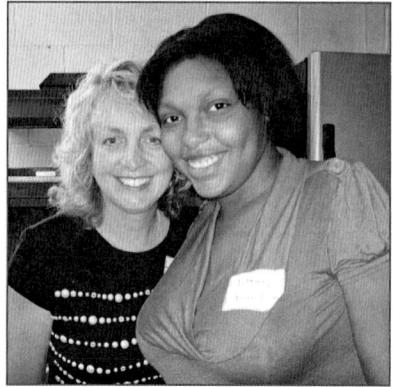

I started Moms2B with Twinkle Schottke by my side. Here we are with our first moms , Cherica Dixon and Tiffany Bailey, in the Grace Missionary Baptist Church in the Weinland Park neighborhood in 2010-11.

As I look back on why, how and with whom we started Moms2B, I realize how far the program has come and I'm heartened by its potential into the future, and beyond our Columbus community. From that first day when Twinkle and I started with just two moms in a church basement in a neighborhood where moms and babies faced so many obstacles to health and well-being, we built something meaningful.

We built it with the community's partnership and the support of many outside organizations and together we made a difference to more than 4,000 moms, babies and families. I'm proud that we made waves in Columbus, Franklin County and the State of Ohio — that we were instrumental in not only supporting moms, babies and families but that we help illuminate the severity of the infant mortality crisis and the disparities that set a treacherous course for Black moms and babies. I will always remember our love and commitment to the pregnant women we served, and hope that love has rippled through to another generation and will persist well into the future. I'm confident that our work helped ensure that babies born to Moms2B attendees felt less stress in the womb and were welcomed by families with more trust that futures could change, families who experienced care and respect during their time in the program.

In writing this book, I've been struck by how many people our group met with — to educate, to learn and to garner support. From ministers to governors, Moms2B staff collaborated with anyone we could to help reduce infant death and support vulnerable moms and babies. We brought in lawmakers, students, nurses, doctors, dietitians, social workers, child development specialists, navigators, community health workers and more, and I'm forever grateful for their openness and contributions. Without this network of advocates, and without Twinkle's unwavering support, energy and smiles, families wouldn't have gained the knowledge, trust, parenting skills and other benefits that we hope helped set them up for success. I believe that those who have been part of Moms2B, or who spent time with us, likely gained empathy and better understanding of the obstacles to good health as well.

For me, to look back on this journey is to see a path full of powerful memories, happy times, critical moments, losses, heartaches, worries, hurdles blocking the path forward, detours, sleepless nights, joy, celebrations, lessons learned and results measured. Many of these memories I tried to faithfully recount in this book.

I tried, with sound advice from Twinkle and from my husband Steve, to leave Moms2B in good hands on a stable foundation with a strong future. I feel confident that Moms2B will remain, though changed, with new leadership, team members and an evolution into a hybrid format with remote teaching and connections.

I believe that the same love, trust and hope that built Moms2B will keep it alive well into the future, supporting moms and families and setting babies on a path to thrive.

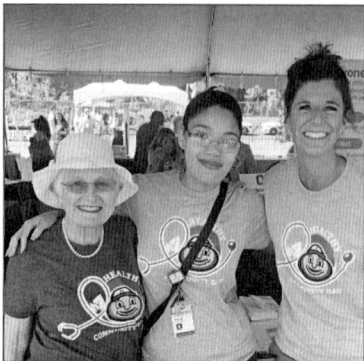

At Ohio State East Hospital on 2022 Community Day with Marriya Roper, a Moms2B navigator and Tabitha Hootman, senior manager.

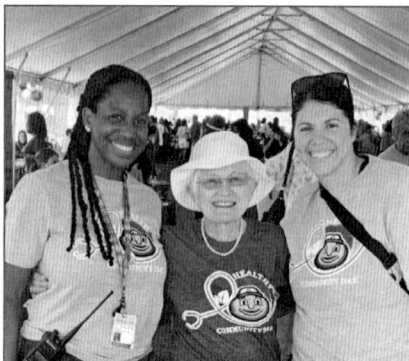

Dr. Kamila Dixon, Moms2B medical director on my right with Annie Marsico from government relations at the Ohio State East Community Day, 2022.

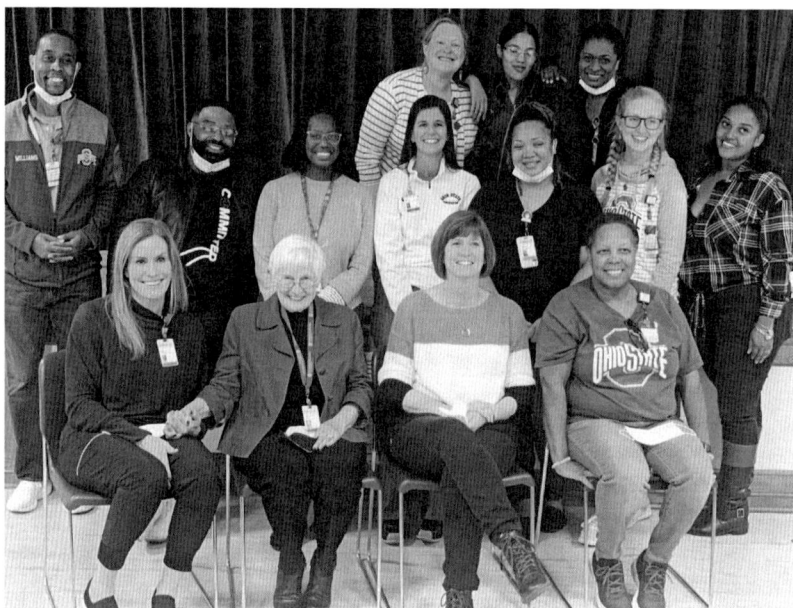

Under new leadership, Steve and I were thrilled to join the Moms2B team at the reopening of in-person sessions at Moms2B East, Oct. 13, 2022.

Chapter References: The Moms2B Story

Introduction

1. Preventing Infant Mortality in Ohio: Task Force Report November 2009 available on-line at the Ohio Department of Health.

Chapter 2. Crime and Protection

2. Felitti VJ, Anda RF, Nordenberg D, Williamson DF, Spitz AM, Edwards V, Koss MP, Marks JS. Relationship of childhood abuse and household dysfunction to many of the leading causes of death in adults. The Adverse Childhood Experiences (ACE) Study. Am J Prev Med. 1998 May;14(4):245-58. doi: 10.1016/s0749-3797(98)00017-8. PMID: 9635069.

3. Lu MC, Halfon N. Racial and ethnic disparities in birth outcomes: a life-course perspective. Matern Child Health J. 2003 Mar;7(1):13-30. doi: 10.1023/a:1022537516969. PMID: 12710797.

Chapter 7. A Time of Growth

4. Desmond, Matthew. 2016 Evicted: Poverty and Profit in the American City. New York: Crown.

5. Gabbe PT, Reno R, Clutter C, Schottke TF, Price T, Calhoun K, Sager J, Lynch CD. Improving Maternal and Infant Child Health Outcomes with Community-Based Pregnancy Support Groups: Outcomes from Moms2B Ohio. Matern Child Health J. 2017 May;21(5):1130-1138. doi: 10.1007/s10995-016-2211-x. PMID: 28074311.

Chapter 10. Key Leaders in Fighting Infant Mortality

6. More information about the Ohio Equity Counties can be found on the Website of City Match-institute-for-equity-in-birth-outcomes and the Ohio Department of Health-Maternal-Infant-Wellness-OEI

7. Dixon-Shambley, K. and Gabbe, P. (2021). Using Telehealth Approaches to Address Social Determinants of Health and Improve Pregnancy and Postpartum Outcomes. Clinical Obstetrics and Gynecology, 64 (2), 333-344. doi: 10.1097/GRF.0000000000000611.

Chapter 12. Moms2B Matters: Measuring our Impact

8. Gabbe PT, Reno R, Clutter C, Schottke TF, Price T, Calhoun K, Sager J, Lynch CD. Improving Maternal and Infant Child Health Outcomes with Community-Based Pregnancy Support Groups: Outcomes from Moms2B Ohio. Matern Child Health J. 2017 May;21(5):1130-1138. doi: 10.1007/s10995-016-2211-x. PMID: 28074311

9. Hade EM, Lynch CD, Benedict JA, Smith RM, Ding DD, Gabbe SG, Gabbe PT. The Association of Moms2B, a Community-Based Interdisciplinary Intervention Program, and Pregnancy and Infant Outcomes among Women Residing in Neighborhoods with a High Rate of Infant Mortality. Matern Child Health J. 2022 Apr;26(4):923-932. doi: 10.1007/s10995-020-03109-9. Epub 2021 Jan 20. PMID: 33471249; PMCID: PMC9052173.

10. Hall ES, Greenberg JM. Estimating community-level costs of preterm birth. Public Health. 2016 Dec; 141:222-228. doi: 10.1016/j.puhe.2016.09.033. Epub 2016 Oct 27. PMID: 27932005.

Acknowledgements

After I decided to retire in June 2021, my husband, Steven Gabbe, encouraged me to write the story of Moms2B and apply to Ohio State's Medical Heritage Center for a George Paulson Scholarship for the support and time I needed. During the months that followed he boosted me over my writing roadblocks and lifted my spirits — along with heavy boxes of files and keepsakes — with love and kindness. He read my drafts and corrected my grammar. With his belief in me and in Moms2B, I wrote this book.

After Steve read my drafts, I sent each chapter to Misti Crane, a former journalist who wrote extensively about infant mortality and later went on to earn her master's degree in public health, conducting research on our graduates as her culminating project. Misti made this book readable and cogent. As a journalist for The Columbus Dispatch, she had covered the Infant Mortality Task Force that I write about in Chapter 8 and produced an award-winning series that helped open the community's eyes to the toll of infant mortality, the roots of disparity and the need for change. The quotes that I use in Chapter 12 come from Moms2B graduates she interviewed for her master's project. They provide more evidence that Moms2B matters. With her deep understanding of the infant mortality crisis in Columbus and her crisp writing style, she helped me deliver on my promise to write this book.

This book describes the program that Twinkle French Schottke and I created together, and I am forever grateful for the once-in-a-lifetime partnership. She brought her irrepressible, uplifting cheerfulness to every session. From pregnancy through birth and infancy she encouraged parents to talk, sing, read and even dance with their infants. She taught how to read infant cues and soften the impact of early trauma. Parents loved it when Twinkle placed infants on quilts to show how to do tummy time, review how and when to introduce food and toys, and taught them what to anticipate next in their child's development.

Together, we recruited a team that reinforced her teachings and made Moms2B successful. Our success would have been impossible without the incredible women we hired early on: Katie Calhoun, Jamie Sager, Carmen Clutter, Tanikka Price, Brandy Warne, Tomassina Richards and Natasha Abrams. Taylor Ollis, Brook Meadows and Lydia Burney joined us later. Over time we hired more nurses, social workers, medical dietitians, navigators and community health workers who brought incalculable contributions to supporting, teaching and building trust with our Moms2B families.

With support from neighborhood churches and their pastors we gained a trustworthy presence in areas with the most need. From opening day in September 2010, Pastor Kevin Miller allowed our team to use Grace Missionary Baptist Church to hold our sessions, our team meetings, and host governors, first ladies, state senators, mayors, students and friends to witness Moms2B in action. Church leaders at five more locations welcomed us in the same generous way: John Edgar and Sue Wolfe at the Church for all People, Keith Troy and Brenda Troy at New Salem Baptist Church, Jennifer Kimball Casto at Epworth United Methodist, Tim Lee at Hillcrest Baptist Church, and Yaves Ellis at New Birth Christian Ministries. With their blessings we gained trust in their neighborhoods, which was reinforced by CelebrateOne, the organization that arose from the Greater Columbus Infant Mortality Task Force to reduce infant mortality rates. Erika Clark Jones, Dawn Tyler Lee and Maureen Stapleton — leaders of that effort — believed in our neighborhood-based group model and further strengthened our relationships in each Columbus neighborhoods we served.

I'm also forever grateful to our volunteers, who expanded the services we could provide at each Moms2B neighborhood session. Many were retired professionals who wanted to give back and help with the infant mortality crisis.

Most have remained loyal contributors for years. Our many student volunteers often used the experience in their personal statements for application to medical school, citing what an important role Moms2B played in their own growth.

I also want to thank the group of team members who, like me, loved the sessions and studied the numbers. They conscientiously collected data and wrestled with databases to create weekly, monthly and, with Becky Reno's help, annual reports that allowed us to collaborate with our research colleagues, Courtney Lynch and Erinn Hade, who studied our outcomes and published findings demonstrating clear evidence that, indeed, Moms2B does save babies!

Adding Dads2B gave us a unique and much needed program, and I'd like to thank David Fluellen and his assistants, especially Louis Pollard. David lived his strong beliefs that fathers need to be responsible and committed to the mothers of their children and parent their children. We owe part of our success to David and Dads2B.

For over a decade the Ohio State Government Relations Office led by Stacy Rastauskas, Jerry Friedman at the Ohio State University Medical Center and his team of Stephanie Milburn, Jenny Carlson, Bill Hayes, Colleen O'Brien and Annie Marsico opened government doors for us to obtain essential funding, including dollars that enabled the expansion to Dayton.

With unwavering support from the Department of Obstetrics and Gynecology, led by Dr. Mark Landon, we found a stable, long-term home. With Mark, Drs. Rebecca Rudesill and Kamilah Dixon, Administrator Kristine Hertl, all of the nurses and physicians at the McCampbell Hall Clinic, and Nurse Manager Anita Cygnor on labor and delivery and postpartum, we have a world class medical team that values Moms2B as an arm of their health care system, reaching into the community to save lives.

Finally, and most importantly, to the more than 4,000 pregnant women and their families who have joined Moms2B over the years, I remain forever grateful for the trust they placed in us. At our first in-person session after the pandemic, a 19-year-old sat in Sister-Brother Circle with his pregnant partner and said, "I came here with my mother when she was pregnant with my little brother. He's nine years old, and now we will have our own Moms2B baby." What a testament to the strength of the program and the families who return to create the next generation of Moms2B babies.

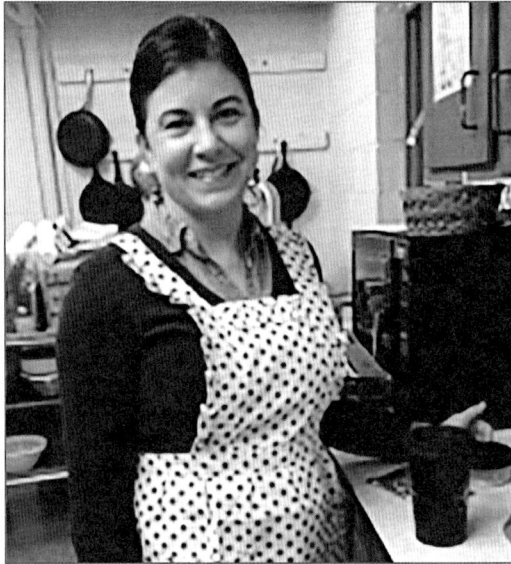

My editor, Misti Crane, in a photo from her volunteer kitchen work at Moms2B in Weinland Park. Thank you Misti for everything!